I0429898

Our Body On Fire

Destroying Our Health

Rudy Kachmann MD

Copyright © 2014 Rudy Kachmann MD
All rights reserved.

ISBN: 1501055747
ISBN 13: 9781501055744

Table of Contents

Preface

WE ARE HAVING A WORLD epidemic of chronic disease, diabetes, heart attacks, strokes, cancer, autoimmune disease and many others.

Our dietary advice was determined by the USDA, NIH, the society of Lung, Heart, and Blood, Ancel Keys, the McGovern commission and the American Heart Association.

For 50 years they said fat was the problem in one form or another. When it was not the fat, it was hydrogenation they recommended, and then it was vegetable oils. All of it made us sick. The obesity rate and chronic disease rate only increased. It's time for change.

This book will explain the history of our chronic disease explosion.

Obesity rates are increasing across the world and so are its secondary consequences. We have a lot of skinny fat people in Asia. They look thin but their metabolism is not right and the rate of type II diabetes is quite high.

Lack of health knowledge is the problem. Sugar causes most of our problems. No wonder we're sick. Our bodies are on fire from the evil twins sucrose and fructose, and their brother omega-6 fat.

In this book we will explain the science to what to do about the problem to make us healthy. We are what we eat and how we think.

History

WE'VE BEEN EXPOSED TO AN avalanche of diets: the Atkins Diet, low carb and high protein, the Paleo diet, also high protein, Pritikin, mostly vegetarian, Dr. Dean Ornish, essentially vegetarian, Dr. Caldwell Esseltyne, Dr. Joel Fuhrman, 80% nutrient dense, 20% low-fat meat products, Dr. Richard Johnson, "The Sugar Fix", "The Rosedale Diet", etc. I've read about them all. Frankly, there's something good in all of them, although I don't agree with everything. There clearly is no "best" diet.

Personally, I think a combination of Dr. Robert Lustig, Dr. Joel Fuhrman, Dr. Caldwell Esseltyne, Dr. Dean Ornish, Dr. Kachmann, my book "Secret of the Non-Diet," and especially Dr. Richard Johnson's book, "The Sugar Fix" and Dr. Ron Rosedale's diet hit the mark. I quote from them liberally.

Dr. Robert Lustig, in his New York Times bestseller "Fat Chance," and Dr. Richard Johnson emphasize the evil twin fructose as the main culprit for our declining health. I agree.

What I witnessed in working at hospitals for 44 years was the horrible complications of vascular disease, heart attacks, strokes, cancer as a result of improper eating and obesity, all of which are incredibly sad. There is great hope because these chronic illnesses are largely preventable and many can be stopped, prevented and reversed. I have seen it. I have taught it!

We need to participate in our healthcare; what we have now is "sick care." We need to speak to our patients, read, research and ask for the help of our families and providers. The wellness wheel begins with participating in your healthcare.

We need to understand the physiology of fructose, what foods contain it and what foods to eat, plus other good health habits like exercise and stress reduction to enjoy a healthy happy life.

In this book you will learn about good carbohydrates, proteins and fats. Yes, fat is not quite the enemy you thought it was, as part of the problem, sugar, is the real toxin.

Twin Metabolism: Glucose and Fructose

THE EVIL TWIN, FRUCTOSE, IS separated from his brother glucose in the gut and heads for the bloodstream. It doesn't raise the insulin level like glucose and without insulin enters the liver cells and starts its evil path of destruction. Fructose, incidentally, is never found in nature without being chemically attached to something else. It's always attached to his brother glucose.

Fructose causes the browning reaction like you see in frying, or what's known as the formation of AGEs, advanced glycation end products.

When glucose attaches to protein in the blood, it can wreak havoc in the body, contributing to aging and chronic disease. The HBA 1C is an example in which we are determining the blood sugar level over a 3-month period. That's why fruit turns brown and becomes a lot sweeter. It's called the Mailard reaction and is 7 times faster than the glucose reaction. This drives the aging process in many degenerative diseases, like arthritis, dementia, cancer, heart disease, breast disease and autoimmune disease.

Fructose leads to inflammation and insulin resistance. The liver metabolizes 95% of fructose and the kidney metabolizes 5%. Let's review the steps of fructose metabolism.

The liver needs 3 times as much energy to metabolize fructose as it does for glucose. Metabolism is defined as the sum of the chemical activity necessary to carry out a reaction. That depletes the level of ATP, adenosine triphosphate, our energy molecule in the mitochondria of our cells. The mitochondria are little energy factories, which every cell has – there are about 10,000 factories per cell, and trillions in the human body. No mitochondria, no energy. The waste product of ATP metabolism is uric acid and purines, which cause hypertension. That's the reason many type 2 diabetics have high blood pressure.

It goes straight to acetyl-coA, exceeding the mitochondria's ability to metabolize it. The acetyl-coA converts the energy of fructose to fat. The fat is deposited mainly in the liver and causes non-alcoholic fatty liver disease, NAFLD. This results in insulin resistance, leptin resistance and inflammation. Leptin is a hormone of fat that regulates fat deposition, appetite and is the king of hormones. If you have leptin resistance, you get fat and it doesn't turn off your appetite like high sugar would without insulin resistance.

Fructose then activates a liver enzyme, which causes inflammation throughout the body, resulting in heart disease, strokes, dementia, cancer and autoimmune disease.

We could not live without glucose. It makes ATP with oxygen, the energy molecule. Twenty percent of our glucose is used for brain fuel, although the brain can use ketones from fat metabolism. Glucose without fructose is called starch, a friendly food source.

When we consume sugar, 20% or so goes to the liver and is converted to glycogen, 80% hits the bloodstream and is utilized for energy by the brain, liver metabolism and muscle.

Glucose metabolism is completely dependent on insulin; it can't enter cells without it. Sugar has a great effect on our brain and some people think it's more addictive than narcotics. Any excess glucose in the liver that's not converted to glycogen or used to create energy will be converted to fat. Yes, glucose and fructose can make you fat; fructose is just a lot worse.

Also glucose can bind to protein, releasing a free radical, an electron, which can destroy your body when in excess. That is called oxidation. It is also called a reactive oxygen species-ROS. They can cause a lot of our chronic diseases and need to be removed.

The History of Glucose and Fructose

AROUND 10,000 YEARS AGO, JUST about when we started agriculture and eventually raising cattle, a plant was discovered in New Guinea called sugarcane. It is a combination of glucose and fructose. All plants produce some sucrose. As a result glucose and fructose are found throughout nature, just different amounts in different plants.

Sucrose is a disaccharide, a combination of 50% each. Lactose is a combination of galactose and glucose. All sugars are sweet, but glucose is 50 to 60% as sweet as fructose. Honey is much sweeter and is 70% fructose. High fructose corn syrup is 55% fructose, 42% glucose. It's a lot sweeter and cheaper.

We are hardwired to seek sugar based on evolution. A survival mechanism. Nature has designed pleasure as a survival mechanism and uses food and sex to do it.

Fruit was probably not cultivated until around 6,000 years ago. Of course the main sugar in fruit is fructose. It is also metabolized in the liver just like the fructose from sucrose.

Our ancestors probably ate 15 to 20 grams of fructose a day. A typical American probably consumes 70-80 grams a day now. Twenty percent of Americans consume 15 to 20% of their diet that way.

Sugarcane spread to Australia, India, Persia and Europe and eventually to Spain and Crete. It was first introduced in England around the year 1000. Christopher Columbus brought sugarcane to Haiti and the Dominican Republic on his second voyage to the New World in 1493. Further, a lot of sugar was imported back to Europe. It started the candy revolution. The Germans in 1747 found that sugar beets were also good source of sugar. Candy bars were sold throughout the 19th century.

Frankly, obesity is probably worse than the plague ever was. The suffering last longer and is now worldwide.

Fructose: The Lipinator

ARE WE THE MOST OBESE nation on earth because of lack of will-power? Other nations think so, but I don't agree. For one thing, many other nations are also becoming overweight. Look at Mexico, which just passed the United States to become the most obese nation on earth. Vietnam and South Korea are running high rates of obesity and type 2 diabetes.

We are programmed through evolution to store energy as a survival mechanism; nature even attached pleasure to it. Food has overpowered us: we don't know how to cook, and glucose and fructose are found throughout our many thousands of processed food items in the food markets. Most are creations of industrial, rather than natural, plants.

Fructose is sweeter than glucose, more tasty, and it offers your brain more reward, turning off the appetite suppressants leptin and ghrelin from your stomach. This means that we might sit down and eat a dozen donuts or a bag of chips. We also know now that fructose depletes your liver of energy, ATP, causes fatty liver and introduces very low density LDL, which is the cause of many health problems.

Eating a high-fat diet can certainly make you fatter if that's a problem to begin with, but the effects of fructose are much more severe.

Fructose fails to satisfy our hunger because it causes leptin resistance, which fails to regulate our fat deposits. We now know that fat is a gland: It is very active, producing hormones, enzymes, cytokines, leptin, etc.

Eating a fructose-rich diet disrupts our metabolism, causing changes in our fat cells. Eating a high fructose diet is one of many ways to increase oxidative stress, a metabolic process related to many diseases. Fructose is 10 times more effective at creating sugar protein products called AGEs, advanced glycation products, which inflame our bodies. Oxidative free radicals are the product of oxygen and sugar metabolism, which is accentuated with fructose metabolism.

Chronic fructose consumption causes insulin resistance, which ends up increasing blood sugar. The sugar attaches to proteins in the blood, resulting in disease and the aging process.

Fructose metabolism is a huge cause of nonalcoholic fatty liver disease (NAFL), cryptogenic cirrhosis, which is the biggest cause of liver transplants. This will be a huge cost to the nation in the future.

Physiology of the Evil Twin and His Brother

JOHN YUDKIN (1910-1995) TRIED TO warn us about sugar. He lost the food fight to Ancel Keys for about 30 years, but his knowledge is now leading the race.

Yudkin, a British physiologist and nutritionist, became internationally famous with his book "Pure, White and Deadly" in 1972. He was one of the first scientists to claim that sugar was a major cause of obesity and heart disease.

I think Dr. Robert H. Lustig, a pediatric endocrinologist from the division of endocrinology at the University of California, San Francisco, has republished Dr. Yudkin's book, as I see his name on the cover. I thank him for that.

For a few decades it was thought that fat was the main culprit in poor health, but the tide is turning.

In his introduction Dr.Lustig says, "Everything old is new again." I was hoping he was talking about me. I'm having my 39th celebration of my 39th birthday next year.

Ancel Keys, the University of Minnesota epidemiologist, stated that saturated fat was the main cause of vascular disease in 1953. He published the 7 countries study.

Dr.Lustig says 3 scientific findings undid the Yudkin case.

By studying the genetic disease of familial hypercholesterolemia, where people at a very young age had very abnormal blood studies, Dr. Michael Brown and Dr. Joseph Goldstein discovered low-density lipoprotein LDL and the LDL receptor, leading to the hypothesis that LDL was the bad actor. We now know that it is very low-density LDL from fructose that is the devil that is killing us. They did not know that at that time and that is what undid Dr. Yudkin. So the fight began and Yudkin was run over by the "fat theory" people. They were wrong.

Additional large studies begin to demonstrate that triglycerides correlated more with sugar consumption. Also, the discovery that very low-density LDL, VLDL was driven by diet, sugar and especially fructose started to change people's thinking about the "fat theory" and Ancel Keys.

Low Carbohydrate Diets

LOW CARBOHYDRATE DIETS CAME TO the forefront, including the Atkins and Paleo diets. In addition, Dr. Raven described Syndrome X, metabolic syndrome.

Dr. Lustig ran across the Yudkin work at a meeting in 2008 and has been a champion ever since (although he was ready doing a great deal of research on sugar and felt it was the real culprit). I think Dr. Lustig is a champion of the sugar fructose debate as well as Dr. Richard Johnson as described in his book "Sugar Fix." They have the answer as far as I'm concerned; I'm just trying to bring the point home because I'm a wellness teacher.

You now know that things have advanced since Dr. Yudkin and the causation is well described by Dr. Richard Johnson and Dr. Lustig. Sugar is addictive and affects the psychology of many people, and it is ruining their health. It affects the serotonin dopamine circuitry of addiction. Dr.Lustig says he is a Yudkin disciple. Put me on the list!

Sugar is the answer to food addiction; if avoided, most people can achieve a normal weight and great health.

The Evil Twin Revisited

DR. YUDKIN, DR. LUSTIG AND DR. RICHARD JOHNSON have advanced the research, education, publication and treatment of chronic disease that is killing us. Many others have written books along the way, including Dr. Dean Ornish, Dr. Joel Fuhrman, Dr. McDougall, Dr. Caldwell Esseltyne of the Cleveland Clinic, Dr. Neal Bernard, Dr. Hans Diehl, and my own books and have helped advance prevention, reversing the treatment of vascular disease, diabetes, cancer prevention, autoimmune disease and more.

The beauty is that the enemy is in our sights and can be killed with one shot: Avoid the evil twin fructose.

Just sit in a restaurant, at a ballgame or school and look at the size of the people. I've been sitting at Starbucks today for more than 2 hours while writing this. The restaurant across the way is even worse. This is a no-judgment zone, but we're not going to solve this problem if we don't really look at it. The same problem is occurring across the world.

In 1890, 5% of Americans were obese. Now it's greater than 35%, plus the 75 to 80% who are overweight. Certain ethnic and racial groups are even approaching 90%.

It's alarming, sickly and costly. Health education is poor; people are eating government-supported genetically altered food. What they do to animals to put them on your plate is beyond comprehension. Milk and cheese products are full of saturated fats, which adds to the problem. Food stamps have no nutrient requirements and are killing people. The poor have a much worse obesity rate because the government-supported food they're eating is influenced by politics and lobbying rather than a focus on good health. Certainly, obesity is psychologically crippling to many people and especially children. A lot of people think it's genetic in origin when it's truly the reaction of the genes to what people are eating. Sometimes a whole family eats the wrong food because they are not aware of what they're doing to themselves, so providers and educators must get more seriously involved.

The government should not support the prices of fat, salt and sugar. They should support organic farming and gardening. I think it's more of what we eat and the amount we are eating. I don't think calorie counting is necessary: Simply eat the right food and exercise 30 minutes a day. We are consuming the evil twin 30% more than in 1970 and that parallels our increase in obesity rates.

Fructose is the main sugar in fruit and has been for 1 million years. Our ancient ancestors and primate animals lived on that. But they exercised a lot and they needed to store fat to survive, so fructose didn't cause the diseases we are seeing.

Some people call high fructose corn syrup "Frankensyrup." It's cheap and sweet and deadly.

In summary, avoiding fructose is a good start on great health. The next few chapters explain how to do it. In addition I would view some other aspects of gluten, which some people are sensitive to as well as saturated fat.

We are FRUCKED

MANY OTHER PRIMATES CAN EXIST on vegetables and fruit alone, have long intestines like us and develop little chronic disease. In nature, fructose intake is limited.

Our ancestors ate only about 20 to 25% fruit in their diet and it was all-seasonal. They did not eat additional sugar like so many of us do today.

Sugar is a big player but the other 50% is fructose, the lion on the field. Sedentary lifestyles and too much animal protein loaded with saturated fat are also a part of the problem. Gluten sensitivity can contribute to this issue and should be tested in everyone.

The White Menace

EVERY SUCCESSFUL DIET RESTRICTS SUGAR, but, as Dr. Lustig says, that is the Lex Luther of the story. Sugar is both a carbohydrate, which a lot of it comes from, as well as a fat, where it can end up if it is not used. These twins, **glucose and fructose,** are the evil ones. Many people are addicted to sugar, and many say that it is as addictive as cocaine.

As already mentioned their chemical formula is the same, but they are metabolized differently.

They affect our mental state by influencing our appetite center, and affect our serotonin and dopamine circuitry. They act like cocaine or heroin and cause the "bliss point" of desire -- the quick fix, the sugar fix. No matter how hard you try, if you don't fix the sugar problem, you won't lose weight. Sugar makes you fat and sick if you consume enough of it

The industrial complex, Cargill, Kellogg, Hershey etc., figured out this bliss point. The Monell Company in Philadelphia, financed by industry and the government studies, knows exactly the amount of sugar and fat it takes to light up our brain with pleasure. They know what foods are most palatable to us. Sales are dependent on it. That's where fast food comes from. They know your bliss point for sugar in adults is 26% and 38% for teenagers. That knowledge is killing us. Children's brains are more easily addicted to sugar, because they're not fully developed.

You've heard of empty calories, calories without nutrients, vitamins, minerals and phytochemicals, and certainly sugar has none of these. Many of us are addicted to sugar but it's the fructose that has a special payload because of its effect on the liver.

Fructose actually is the main sugar in fruit, which we all know, that is good for us! Wrong! In reasonable quantities, consumed in its original form, with fiber and no more than 35 grams daily, it's quite healthy. Fruit juice has more fructose than high fructose corn syrup. But fructose in fruit is not that metabolically different from the fructose and sucrose in corn syrup, to my dismay. To my surprise, excess fruit consumption can have its problems, too. We prefer fructose because it is sweet, it hits the bliss point.

Industry knows how to make it from corn syrup, and recognized that it is sweeter than regular sucrose and cheaper, making a lot of money because of it. Just read the book "Fat, Salt and Sugar" by reporter Michael Moss. High fructose corn syrup was invented by the Japanese in the late 1960s and its consumption has skyrocketed. Today, it is at least 50 to 75% of the cause of our obesity and chronic disease problems. Just look around in a public place, it's plain scary. Many people think this epidemic is genetic when actually it is the reaction of our bodies to the sugar epidemic.

We consume 6.5 ounces of sugar a day, and 130 pounds a year, including about 50 pounds of fructose yearly. We have increased our fructose consumption 5-fold in 100 years. The CDC says 50% of us are consuming at least one fructose drink a day, and 10% drink 3 or more daily.

Sugar has infiltrated thousands of manufactured foods we see in the major markets. Much of our consumption actually comes from manufactured food combinations, and 20% of our calories come from sugar products. We consume 20 teaspoons full of sugar daily. Some of our teenagers are consuming 30 to 40% of their calories from sugar. It's occurring all over the world.

I read in the newspaper the other day that Mexico just surpassed us in obesity, which puts us in the number 2 spot in the western world. They imposed a 10% sales tax on sugary sodas, and an 8% tax on fast food. From what I know about the economic formula called the elasticity of demand that will not change the behavior of the people, although it's a good start. Vietnam, South Korea and Asia are all reporting high rates of type 2 diabetes and obesity. Many have restaurants with the same name and you can see the problem. Fat, salt and sugar. The global consumption of sugar has increased 50%.

The American Heart Association recommends 150 sugar calories a day for men and 100 calories a day for women, but we are blowing past that at around 500-600 calories.

We'd all like to blame high fructose corn syrup as being the main devil, but actually that is only partially true. Fructose is fructose, yes, even from fruit. Fiber keeps us from absorbing some of the sugar, but fructose is still fructose.

High fructose corn syrup consumption is going down because of government laws, but it's a public health problem and we need stronger national laws. At least we have started to control trans-fats and we could do the same for fructose by limiting it. Meanwhile, obesity rate continues to increase. It's the "evil twin" at work.

My friend Dr. Joel Fuhrman was hired to teach proper nutrition in South Korea because of the obesity and type 2 diabetes problem. He told me all about it when I was with him in Italy recently.

Dr. Robert Lustig says in his famous book "Fat Chance" that scientific evidence supports the notion that HFCS is actually no different from sucrose, although high fructose corn sugar does generate a higher blood fructose level, which could have metabolic consequences. But the difference is small, 10 to 15%.

Dr. Lustig says that sugar in any form is toxic. I say fructose is just the evil twin of its malignant brother, glucose. All sugar is potentially toxic and I completely agree with Dr. Lustig. Calorie for calorie, orange juice is worse for you than soda. Orange juice has 1.8 grams of fructose; soda has 1.7 g of fructose, according to Dr.Lustig.

Sugar

SUGAR IS OUR COCAINE. WE are hardwired for sweets by evolution. All our survival instincts like sex and eating are attached by chemistry to pleasure. Sugar makes us feel great and is addictive.

Our taste buds for sugar are located throughout the mouth, tongue, hard palate, and soft palate and down the esophagus to the stomach and even beyond to the pancreas and bowel. Sugar receptors have been found throughout this region. The receptors are not located just on the tip of the tongue, as some people might want to make you think. We have taste for salt, sugar, bitter and sour, and appreciate the softness and palatability of fat although no receptors have been found for fat. It is thought that there is a sense of taste for meat products called umami. We have thousands of taste bud receptors for sugar and they're hooked to the brain, the pleasure center.

As you know sugar is in a lot of our drinks, causing at least one half of the obesity epidemic, and is an ingredient in 80% of all 60,000-food products. Our sugar comes from 3 products: cane sugar, sugar beets and corn.

Christopher Columbus brought sugar to the New World and it was planted in Santo Domingo. The Germans discovered in the 1700s that you could extract glucose from beets. People in France realized you could extract sugar from beets during wartime and now it's grown that way all over the world. Beets were the main source of sugar around 1970. Then the Japanese invented high fructose corn syrup, HFCS, which is much sweeter and cheaper and became very popular in the industry quickly. One of the reasons that it's cheaper is because the U.S. government supports the price of corn.

Unfortunately, corn syrup is high in fructose, which is not metabolized in the bloodstream but metabolized in the liver and made into low density LDL, the one that doesn't float and burrows its way into the blood vessels, neural cells and so on; it also has a lot to do with arthritis and hypertension.

In the 1960s it was proven in lab rats that sugar is addictive. Graduate student Anthony Scalafani studied the effectiveness of sugar and fat with functional MRI scans. The brain just lit up. He published a paper in 1976 with experimental proof of food craving as an addiction.

In Philadelphia there is a place called the Monell Chemical Senses Center, which is supported 50% by the government and 50% by the food industry. Guess who has a lot of influence there? They found and discovered a blood protein that is on the taste buds for sugar. That's how they were able to trace the tremendous distribution of sugar taste buds throughout the mouth, esophagus and gut.

They also determined that children and African-Americans were particularly keen on foods that are salty and sweet. The marketing people have taken full advantage of that. Hypertension is particularly high in the African-American population, so salt intake turns out to be something they really have to watch. When I worked in Washington D.C. as a resident in neurosurgery, I treated a lot of brain hemorrhages from hypertension in the black population. I saw blood pressures that were so high that I've never seen again, fortunately.

At the Monell Institute, they proved that children were actually becoming addicted to sugar because they were developing a tolerance for sugar. In other words you had to keep on increasing the amount, just like a narcotic addict, to get the same effect.

It's the taste, the flavor, the sensation and the psychological satisfaction that they are looking for.

Babies are born with taste buds for sugar and it's based on their biology, it's based on evolution and it's important for the survival.

A man named Moscowitz from White Plains, New York, whose company dealt with product development related to food substances and chemicals, did his best work with sugar. He used mathematical calculations to create the biggest crave. Moscowitz worked on "optimal sensory linking." Hunger was found to be a poor driver of cravings. Emotional needs are more important.

Taste, aroma, appearance and texture are very important.

The convenience of fast food restaurants brought the fat and sugar chemicals to the forefront of the etiology of obesity. The "cocaine effect" of sugar is its mother and father. The king is sugar because of fructose. Convenient, fast and addictive, salt and sugar drive the car. That process has been experimentally, chemically and mathematically proven. Look at the result: America the land of obesity.

It all started at the beginning of the last century. John Harvey Kellogg took over a health facility in Battle Creek, Michigan. The popular diagnosis at that time was neurasthenia and he ran a 400-bed hospital or institute. He came back from a trip to Colorado with an idea to create a breakfast cereal from corn. His brother Will, the accountant, managed to figure out how to make the cereal sweeter and the rest is history.

Fat-laden breakfast foods of the 1900s were then replaced by the sugar-laden cereals of the 20th century and we've all seen the result. Kellogg was home to 108 brands of cereal, and he then developed his own company doing the same thing. Kellogg was composed of the top players for a long time.

The FDA was in bed with these companies and didn't consider sugar as being a threat to our health.

Dr. Jean Mayer, a Harvard professor, called obesity the disease of civilization. He discovered that the desire to eat was controlled by the hypothalamus in the brain.

Advertising to small children by food companies became rampant. They outlawed it in European countries. We restricted it only up to age 11 after a long fight, but companies simply increased advertisements to teenagers, and sales were not affected much.

Robert Woodruff, the CEO of Coke, had 2 brilliant but deadly innovations. In 1927 he introduced Coke with its sugary drinks to the rest of the world; in World War II any soldier anywhere in the world could get a Coke for 5 cents. I suspect he addicted the whole bunch. He figured out how to get into people's emotions with sugar.

A man named Jeffrey Dunn became head of the South American division of Coke; in 2001 he visited Brazil looking for new territory. He was looking at poor neighborhoods for the potential of sales. He woke up and said, "I'm not going to do this." He decided the company went too far. Guess what? He no longer worked for Coke after that trip.

The Coke and Pepsi war has sugar as its king, with coffee not far behind.

In 1981 Coca Cola switched to fructose corn syrup because it was cheaper and sweeter; when they studied their customer base they didn't speak about loyal customers but called them heavy users, like you speak about a drug addict.

Eighty percent of world sugar is consumed by 20% of the people.

Nestlé, Kraft, Coke and Pepsi all decreased the size of the drinks for a while so they could charge less and increase sales, especially in countries like Brazil. It's called the elasticity of demand. I see it demonstrated at my gym and it works. They have 9,000 members where I work out, $10 a month, I compliment them every day. A lot of people are getting in shape there. What they don't realize, though, is exercise is only about 25% of it.

I noticed in the news that Mexico may be passing a law putting a 10% tax on sugars and soda and 8% on fast food. Hallelujah to that.

In 1964, a man named John Yudkin published a book in Britain called "Pure, White and Deadly." He also published countless papers on the biochemistry of sucrose. Remember sucrose is 50% glucose, 50% fructose. Fructose gives the sweetness, is metabolized by the liver and converted to low-density cholesterol, small LDL fragments that penetrate the blood vessels and cause atherosclerosis and a number of other illnesses. It's clearly a toxin and is associated with vascular disease, heart disease, strokes, and other inflammatory illnesses.

Ancel Keys, an epidemiologist from Minnesota, invented the K rations used during the Second World War. However, people started to note that high-fat dishes were leading to a high rate of vascular disease. This resulted in a battle between the fat and sugar camps as to the cause of disease.

In 1970, Michael Brown and Joseph Goldstein in Dallas discovered the HDL, LDL cholesterol and described the LDL receptor. This was a very important discovery. They correlated LDL-cholesterol with coronary heart disease.

Then we followed through with a national low-fat diet recommendation and forgot about the sugar.

Sen. George McGovern appointed a reporter named Nick Mottern with no scientific background to research and write a paper called the "dietary goals for the US." He gathered information from the work of Mark Hegsted at Harvard, a nutritionist. The latter thought that saturated fat was the cause of our health problems. The USDA, the American Heart Association and the Society of Clinical Nutritionists all endorsed the document.

The industry responded with low-fat, high-sugar products and you can see the result. A very obese nation became worse.

The mistake was in assuming that all LDL was bad; it turns out there are 2 types of LDL, A and B. As already mentioned, the large LDL floats in the blood vessels and represents 80% of it. Of the small LDL, 20% is produced in the liver by glucose and fructose, not fat.

A nurse's health study followed 50,000 nurses that were postmenopausal and fed them a 30% fat diet versus 40% fat and they found no difference in the incidence of vascular disease. I've heard others say that they didn't drop it low enough and that's a justifiable criticism. Dr. Joel Fuhrman said they should've dropped to 20% and the results would have been different.

The food industry took the fat out. The food tasted like cardboard and they solved that problem quickly by adding a lot of sugar. Sales went up tremendously and the industry was very happy and the country became sick. Our federal government supported the price of corn, wheat and rye. In the 1990s more low-fiber and high-sugar foods were produced. The obesity epidemic was born.

Seemingly logical, well-meaning people who don't under-stand the biochemistry of food have made a lot of people sick and continue to do so.

Our bodies have not adjusted to all of this sugar, especially fructose, and it's killing us; we consume 60 pounds of fructose a year, 33 pounds of high-fat cheese, 150 pounds of sugar. We are sugar and fat loaded; nobody and our bodies are revolting.

It's become a public health problem and the government needs to act.

Metabolic Syndrome

METABOLIC SYNDROME IS ALSO CALLED insulin resistance syndrome or Syndrome X. To make a diagnosis, you need to consider a number of risk factors.

In 2005, the American Heart Association and the National Heart, Lung and Blood Institute published the following risk profile for metabolic syndrome:

- Is your HDL number below 40 for men or below 50 for women?
- Are your triglycerides over 150?
- Is your waist size 35 inches or above for women, or 40 inches or above for men?
- Are you a pre-diabetic or diabetic, with fasting glucose 100 or greater?
- Is your blood pressure consistently 130/85 or greater?

Metabolic syndrome is a combination of multiple cardiac risk factors believed to be a product of insulin resistance. Our cells, protected by receptors, control which nutrients are allowed in. If the receptors on the cells are made sticky, then the insulin cannot transport the sugar into the cell and that is what we called insulin resistance.

Unfortunately, these receptors can become resistant to insulin's action, probably as a result of weight gain and physical inactivity. This scenario, if repeated over time, is thought to trigger a series of metabolic maladies culminating in metabolic syndrome.

The condition directly damages the coronary arteries, causing the build-up of plaque and promoting blood clots.

Metabolic syndrome affects more than 75 million Americans. It was originally described by Dr. Gerald M. Raven at Stanford University and he called it Syndrome X. Insulin resistance is at the crossroads of this X with obesity, hypertension, abnormal blood fats and high triglycerides being the 4 legs.

Frankly, you can generally look at a person and guess whether they have metabolic syndrome by their body size. Actually, about 20% of people with metabolic syndrome or syndrome X are of normal weight but their blood factors are abnormal. So it is important to get your lipid profile, CRP, and other indicators of inflammation. Many providers use only 2 or 3 of these indicators to make a diagnosis. This improves the chances of reversing the condition.

Insulin resistance is the key to the diagnosis. Insulin is one of the body's most powerful hormones, a class of chemicals that cause enormous physiological changes. It can cause inflammation of the joints that lead to arthritis and also can cause sodium retention in our body, resulting in hypertension, and type 2 diabetes, dementia, etc.

Many people walking around with metabolic syndrome have been totally undiagnosed. This is extremely serious because with proper treatment, they could prevent the development of serious chronic diseases and avoid a lot of suffering, medical costs and possibly disability and death. Many go blind, need to have transplants and even have extremities amputated. There is a much higher rate of dementia and Alzheimer's disease also among these patients. These "skinny-fat" patients are of normal weight but have metabolic syndrome – many are Asians!

It is my opinion and the opinion of many others that the most accurate test to determine insulin resistance is the 2-hour glucose tolerance test. But it is critical to test blood sugar as well as the serum insulin. Stage one is insulin resistance. Also, I suggest the HbA1c but it may be normal because the blood sugar was not elevated. It is critical to know your insulin level, which many times is forgotten and not commonly ordered.

The shape of the body can also give you clues as to insulin resistance in metabolic syndrome. Apple shape is more threatening than pear-shaped, since this type of person generally has more fat inside the liver, pancreas or intestines. Subcutaneous fat is not as threatening, as seen in a pear-shaped individual.

A person under a lot of stress would tend to have a big belly because of steroids, specifically cortisol, which like to deposit fat there; that also is a sign of insulin resistance and pre-diabetes or diabetes.

Very low-density cholesterol (VLDLDL) is the most dangerous of the fats because it can inflame your arteries and damage the endothelium, resulting in invasion of the endothelium by fat deposits.

Insulin also turns on the sympathetic nervous system, your stress response system, resulting in elevation of the blood pressure, your general stress reaction and also increased sugar and fat metabolism.

In 1997 the federal government recommended that all people should be checked for diabetes by age 45. It's my opinion that a lot of these diabetic patients are being missed because they don't get the proper tests.

A national survey revealed in 1998 that the baby boomers are being diagnosed with pre-diabetes at age 37. In 1998 the CDC recommended that every adult be checked for diabetes by age 25. I say let's try age 15 or less because of the great number of obese teenagers.

The earlier we make a diagnosis, the sooner we can begin to avoid a lot of chronic disease; we could turn this into the healthiest nation in the world and improve our ranking of 37 according to the World Health Organization at this time.

Liquid White Gold

COCA-COLA WAS DISCOVERED IN A pharmacy in Atlanta in 1886 and started a revolution in sugary products. In 1968, it was discovered that if you took an enzyme called glucose isomerase, you could make corn syrup a lot sweeter and cheaper because the government was supporting the price of corn. In 1971 the Japanese discovered a way of converting the sugar in corn syrup to fructose and the rest is history.

Fructose increases the shelf life of processed foods, makes food cheaper and sweeter, increases the rate of sugar joining up with proteins in the blood, which increases the rate of aging and is the cause of a lot of diseases including dementia. It also affects the brain, increasing appetite.

In the 1950s, '60s and '70s, Dr. Cleve and Dr. Yudkin proposed the sugar theory of disease, but they were thrown under the bus for 30 years by the "fat theory" as the cause of obesity and chronic disease. The latter is being disproven at this time. Be sure to read Dr. Richard Johnson's "Sugar Fix" and "Fat Change," and Dr. Richard Lustig's "Fat Chance."

Our genetic structure has changed very little in the last hundred thousand years. Food is information, and our bodies are revolting against the new foods, resulting in chronic diseases.

The Master Disease of Our Time: Sugar Addiction

THE GREEKS SPOKE ABOUT THE mythological giant, Anteus, who became stronger whenever he touched his mother, the earth. He was conquered by Hercules when he held him off the ground.

2500 years later, we have been lifted off the earth by the modern industrial complex. We have been held captive by the power of the industrial complex and the government. It's a world of thousands of processed food items made in a plant, along with their accompanying hormones, pesticides, herbicides and genetically altered food that is killing us.

Dr. Norman Cleve, who had been the chief medical officer of a battleship in WWII, was the first to propose that taking off the germ and the bran resulted in a sugary product that caused most of Western diseases. He set out the concept that most Western diseases were caused by consuming refined carbohydrate foods.

He felt the fundamental problem lay in the fact that Westerners had a profound change in their diet in a very short period of time, which did not allow for evolutionary adaptation. Dr. D. P. Burkett from England, also way ahead of his time, agreed with that. Dr. Robert Lustig also agrees. The mass incrimination of sugar and white flour as the cause of a lot of Western diseases was first advanced by Dr. Cleve in 1956.

Dr. Cleve used the term "the saccharine disease" and published that book in 1956, so I think we may need to give them the original credit for this concept.

He also stresses the term "simplicity," reminding us that the biggest advances in humanity have been simple. He called saccharine a refined carbohydrate in that it caused a carbohydrate disease.

No distinction between the twins, glucose and fructose, and especially the evil twin fructose, was made because the science had not advanced far enough. The metabolism of fructose was likely not known at that time. Let's face it, the chemical formula for **glucose** and fructose is the same, fructose is just an isomer of glucose. Another simple explanation: High fructose corn syrup had not been invented yet either.

Dr. Cleve brings up Charles Darwin's law of adaptation. He states that there hasn't been enough time in terms of evolution for our bodies to adapt to this onslaught of new processed food.

Both Dr. Cleve and Dr. Yudkin thought that sugar was the cause of the majority of Western diseases. Dr. Cleve thought that removing fiber exposed the carbohydrates' endosperm, causing constipation, varicose veins, diverticulitis, cancer of the colon, dental disease, type 2 diabetes, obesity, vascular disease, heart attacks and strokes.

Dr. Cleve also spoke about change in our intestines, and how 500 different bacteria and viruses living there can result in a significant amount of disease.

We know of Dr. Ancel Keys entering the picture in the '50s and the studies he did in the Mediterranean area. He proposed that fat causes chronic Western diseases and eventually Dr. Cleve and Dr. Yudkin were thrown under the bus for 30 years.

But now we have defined fructose, and its metabolic effects on the liver, as a cause of Western diet-induced diseases. The real evil twin fructose has been discovered and we now know what he looks like in spite of having the same chemical configuration as glucose, $C_6H_{12}O_6$, but the atoms are arranged differently.

High Fructose Corn Syrup (HFCS)

THE "BLISS POINT" FOR PLAIN old sugar as you might suspect has been found by the food manufacturers: It's 26% for adults, and 36% for children. In other words, as adults, if 26% of our food is sugar, it would still be palatable. Sales were becoming stagnant so the industry needed something sweeter and especially cheaper.

In 1970 the Japanese invented high fructose corn syrup (HFCS). It is now made from government-supported corn; the sugar from corn syrup is modified with an enzyme and that makes it a lot sweeter and cheaper. Unfortunately, it's metabolized differently, and was placed in soft drinks and a lot of other foods. Some restrictions have been made in certain states to restrict the sale because of health hazards. Then again, it is not that different from regular sucrose, which is 50% of glucose and 50% sucrose. Certainly, Dr. Robert Lustig, a pediatric endocrinologist, thinks so and put that on his "YouTube DVD" and his great book called "Fat Chance." He hit the nail on the head as to the cause of our obesity epidemic.

It is my opinion, well supported in the literature and my books plus 44 years of experience, that sugar is a toxin that makes us sick and fructose is the "Evil Twin." Remember sucrose and table sugar is 50% glucose and 50% fructose.

Sugar is both a carbohydrate and a fat and I will prove it to you.

Sugar is bar none the most successful food additive.

Now, because of fructose corn syrup, which is so much cheaper, sugar in some form is found in 80% of our 60,000 food products.

Sugar is made from 50% glucose and 50% fructose. It's fructose that makes it sweet, that is the molecule we want. It's fructose that causes metabolic syndrome and accompanying diseases. The changes occur in the liver because that is where fructose is metabolized.

After digestion, the sugar molecule splits into sucrose and fructose. Fructose goes straight to the liver and is rapidly converted to fat and not used for energy. Of the 50% of the sucrose that is sugar, only 25% goes to the liver versus 80% of the fructose which heads straight for the liver and is converted to low density LDL, the nasty stuff that causes vascular disease. Glucose can replace your glycogen stores, your sugar stores that are used widely for exercise and daily activity.

Americans consume 150 pounds of sugar yearly, 6.5 ounces a day. Our consumption has doubled in 30 years. The CDC estimates that Americans consume one can of sweetened drink daily; 5% consume 4 drinks a day. World consumption has doubled in 50 years.

The American Heart Association recommends only 200 calories from sugar per day and that is being exceeded all over the world.

The fructose corn syrup consumption rate has gone down a bit because of education and the change of some laws in cities like New

York. Mayor Michael Bloomberg has done his best but he didn't get everything done that he wanted to do in that direction. Except from fruit because of its fiber, fructose is toxic and is killing a lot of us. Incidentally, the fructose in fruit is metabolically no different!

Orange juice is worse than fructose corn syrup: In just one eight-ounce glass, there are nearly 2 grams of fructose. The same thing goes with soda.

All sweets have fructose, including white sugar, beans, table sugar, honey, brown sugar, etc.

Sugar stimulates our serotonin and dopamine circuitry and makes us feel good quickly. A significant number of us, including newborns, are addicted to sugar. The bigger you are, the more likely that has occurred; you may not even be aware of it. Sugary drinks account for 50% of the obesity in the United States and the world over. Diet drinks aren't much better because they have a sweet taste that encourages people to eat more sugary foods and the obesity epidemic continues.

Certainly, if you're an athlete in the middle of a major event and drinking sugary drinks, you would probably get away with it because you are using them up as energy very quickly, but the rest of us watching the race will gain weight quickly although fructose is not metabolized quickly.

When the fructose is metabolized in the liver and causes insulin resistance, it does not turn off our appetite or signal the brain that we have enough energy and so it leads to weight gain. That is because of leptin and insulin resistance.

Our bodies have not adjusted to the sugary glut and we gain weight instead and develop insulin resistance, type 2 diabetes and many other chronic illnesses.

As already mentioned, sugar is added to about 80% of our 60,000 foods and we don't even notice it, so reading labels becomes important. The government supports the price of sugar, which is making us sick; it supports the price of corn, the source of fructose corn syrup; your own government has declared war on you. The lobbyists for these food companies pass out a lot of money to the politicians whose main concern appears to be to be reelected and your health is irrelevant. They can show us the food plate all they want, but actions speak louder than words. We lead the world in vascular disease, diabetes, cancer and autoimmune disease. Remember the critical worlds: Sugar is 50% fructose, it's a carbohydrate and a fat and that's what's killing us. Read your labels, talk to the waiter, always ask where the food came from. You need to be an informed consumer or you'll surely get sick.

What is inflammation?

WHEN I SEE AN OVERWEIGHT or obese person, I see a fire. We have 300,000 miles of blood vessels and 600,000 miles of lymphatic vessels, twice that of our vascular system.

When you consume a large amount of fructose, the other 50% of sucrose, table sugar, yes the same sugar as in fruit, bodies become inflamed. You don't see the fire because it is low-grade; it is hidden in your body, mostly. Although, it can be visible in your skin as advanced wrinkling as you might see in a smoker or a person with a chronic disease like type II diabetes.

You don't develop symptoms immediately as if your house was burning down, it's a long-term process.

Presenting as vascular disease, blindness, retinopathy, neuropathy, amputations, renal disease, renal transplants, many types of cancer and autoimmune diseases, this fire is a serious burn.

Inflammation is an attempt by the body to heal itself, so it's not all bad, the trouble that it's overdoing it.

Anytime a virus, bacteria or a foreign protein, a toxin invades your body, the Army, Navy, Air Force and Marines go to work to defend you, increasing blood flow to the site of the fire or infection. .

Other times the body essentially is attacking itself, increasing the chance of developing autoimmune diseases like lupus, rheumatoid arthritis and some demyelinating neurological diseases.

This thin layer lining of blood vessels called endothelium becomes inflamed by a nano-sized lipoprotein produced in the liver by fructose, resulting eventually in the buildup of arterial plaque. An essential fatty acid called omega-6 produced by vegetable oils, nonorganic raised beef, and farm-raised fish can do the same thing. The fructose were eating, though, is the main culprit.

Fructose appears to set the stage for the formation of several metabolic activities.

When you consume fructose, it can inflame your gut, even punch holes in your gut resulting in inflammation. It then enters the bloodstream and does not raise your insulin level, so it doesn't turn your appetite off, goes to the liver and activates the fructose enzyme, rapidly uses your energy molecule, ATP, and produces fat in your liver, resulting eventually in non-alcoholic fatty liver disease. At least 25% of Americans have non-alcoholic fatty liver disease and are not aware of it. They may even be of normal weight and their blood work is off. For example, the CRP, C-reactive protein may be elevated on a blood test. Fructose stimulates the production of uric acid. Uric acid directly induces inflammation in your arterial system. Fructose causes a low-grade infection and the first symptom is inflammation, which can go on for many years, gradually causing serious diseases.

Chronic inflammation is a serious problem with far-reaching consequences for your health.

A Calorie in is Not a Calorie out!

GLUCOSE IS A FORM OF energy you were designed to run on. Every cell in your body, every area and in fact every little thing on earth uses glucose for energy.

If you receive fructose only from vegetables and fruits as most people did a century ago, you would consume about 15 grams per day, a far cry from the 73 grams per day the typical adolescent consumes from sweetened drinks. In vegetables and fruits, fructose is mixed with fiber, vitamins, minerals, enzymes and beneficial phyto-nutrients, all of which moderate any negative metabolic effects.

It isn't the fructose itself that is bad; it's the massive dose most people consume that makes it dangerous.

Your body metabolizes fructose in a much different way than glucose. The entire burden of metabolizing fructose falls on your liver. People are consuming fructose in enormous quantities, which has made the negative effects much more profound. Today, 55% of sweeteners used in food and beverage manufacturing are made from corn, and the number one source of calories in America is soda, in the form of high fructose corn syrup.

The troops

YOUR ARMY, NAVY, MARINES AND Air Force are activated by eating food, which is genetic information, and may not be compatible with your genetic structure. The majority of what we are eating is a new invention; the genetic structure of food has been changed very rapidly. Ten thousand years is not enough time to cause a significant change in our genes and DNA and our bodies are revolting and making us sick.

The B-lymphocytes of your lymphatic system produce a defending army of antibodies trying to fight off the invaders of newly invented or over-consumed foods. Like the evil twins, sugar, fructose and omega-6's. The neutrophils are the Marines attacking the inflammatory process itself. The macrophages are part of the lymphatic system that acts like the garbage collector. They take advantage of our 600,000 miles of lymphatic vessels in attempt to clean up the body. That's why a lymphatic massage makes us feel better.

The T lymphocytes are the storm troopers that invade the body outside the blood vessels and lymphatic system and try to heal us!

The defending army is aided by fatty acids called leukotriene's and prostaglandins made from fatty acids called arachidonic acid.

These are our essential fatty acids that we need to consume and are not made by the body. Remember, not all fats are bad.

Swelling and redness indicate inflammation. Prostaglandins help form that and also dilate the local capillaries to increase the blood flow to the area. They also stimulate nerve fibers and secrete chemicals that cause pain and point out the problem. That's acute inflammation, what we have is chronic inflammation accompanied by very little pain unless it's in a very advanced condition although skin changes can occur early on. Smokers for example may look 20 years older than they really are, and type II diabetes often have similar cosmetic changes.

Aspirin and ibuprofen can block the prostaglandin's effect but can have their own complications, including excessive bleeding or inability to clot.

How does inflammation become disease?

THE INFLAMMATORY PROCESS IS TRYING to aid us, but on a chronic basis it may be overdoing it. **The body** thinks it's defending us, but instead is attacking itself.

When very low density LDL inflames our vascular system, it occurs throughout the whole body, more so in some areas than others. Many diabetics have problems with vision, numbness in their hands and feet, hypertension and increased incidence of heart attacks and strokes. Memory loss is rampant. That's why I'm trying to prevent and treat this chronic disease very early in its process. We could prevent most of that. Most people do not even know that type II diabetes is preventable in a few weeks or months a good 90% of the time. The reaction is like putting a blowtorch to light candles on the birthday cake, easy does it, but that is not what is happening.

Patients with chronic inflammatory disease many times need knee and hip replacements. The main cause is not that they weigh a lot, some actually don't, it's the inflammation of the joints caused by the combination of sugar and proteins plus insulin.

If you want to know the rate your body is aging, get an HVA1C test, which tests your blood sugar over the last 3 months. It's a combination of sugar and proteins in your blood. That test is best to determine your rate of aging. Inflammation is also a big cause of cancer, autoimmune diseases, like lupus and arthritis of the knees and hips. Type II diabetics often need hip and knee replacements because of this.

The Good Fats

YES, WE HAVE SOME GOOD fats, and they are essential for our existence.

They have been with us since the beginning of time. They are called essential fatty acids, have to be consumed as food, and we could not live without them.

Millions of years ago before we developed a circulatory system, we used fatty acids as communicators, like the internet; they were then and still are today our basic communicating system between our 70 trillion cells. They are rapidly made and destroyed making them difficult to study. They were first identified in the prostate gland, which is why you hear the term prostaglandins; you have to collect thousands of animal prostate glands just to have a few for study.

The essential fats omega-3 and omega-6 are converted through enzymatic processes to various other fatty acids like EPA, DHA and the anti-inflammatories and the pro-inflammatory AA arachidonic acid, prostaglandins, thromboxane and leukotriene's. Our ancient ancestors ate a ratio of omega-3 versus omega-6 of about 2:3. We are now eating omega-6's 20/1 over omega-3s. We are indeed inflamed. We are on fire. That's why we see so much advanced disease, heart disease, strokes, cancer, autoimmune disease, dementia and more.

The pro-inflammatory fatty acids are found in animal products, genetically modified corn, high fructose corn syrup and cattle from concentrated animal feeding organizations as well as pond-raised fish. When eating or shopping out, always ask - where did this beef or fish come from? That's why it is important to eat organic raised beef, lamb, pork and fish.

Things got a lot more interesting though when Dr. Bang and Dr. Dyerberg from Denmark went to Greenland and studied the Eskimos. At that time there was a lot of nasty disease and diabetes in Denmark, but they had heard that the Eskimos were eating a very high-fat diet but had little evidence of heart attacks, strokes and cancer. This work was done in the 1960s and 1970s.

The Eskimos were eating a 50% fat diet of blubber from seals and whales and had little evidence of heart disease, vascular disease and diabetes.

In 2003 we switched from a low-fat regimen to high-fat diet. The Atkins diet became the rage. We followed the advice of Dr. Ancel Keys for 30 years and become sicker every year. About 50% of people now have diabesity and we are heading even higher.

The first of omega-3s - ALA, a-linolenic acid, is the parent of these fatty acids. They are found mainly in the leaves of plants and other green parts of the plants. They are associated with the photosynthetic process of plants. Yes, plants have some fat in them; even though it is not very much per plant, it is the most prevalent essential fatty acid in the universe considering the pure volume of plant structures.

One glycerol and 3 fatty acids make one triglyceride, your fat molecule.

DHA, Dehydroascorbic acid, is a child of alpha-linolenic acid. DHA is used by humans and animals for vision, thinking, nerve conduction and is a fast moving fatty acid. It is related to the structure of the fatty acid. These essential fatty acids move very quickly and have a short lifespan. DHEA is the quick-change artist. Your brain is full of DHEA.

Alpha-linolenic acid is found in the chloroplasts of plants, the green part. It is the most abundant fat on earth. DHA and EPA accumulate in animals because they eat the plants. Deficiencies of EPA, DHA, have resulted in a host of human illnesses including vascular disease; type 2 diabetes, cancer, dementia, etc.

DHA needs to be in our eyes, brain, heart and all other tissues. That's why ocean fish and some omega-3 supplements, like EPA, ALA and DHA have value.

DHA was not the first of omega-3s discovered; that was EPA-Eicosapentaenoic acid. It has 20 carbon atoms, eikosi means 20 in Greek.

These were discovered by the 2 Danish physicians, Dr. Bang and Dr. Dyerberg, who studied the Eskimos in Greenland in the 1970s. They studied the Eskimos and their blood with gas-liquid-chromatography, a fairly new invention.

They published a paper in the journal *Lancet* suggesting that the explanation for the Eskimos' longevity and lack of disease was the consumption of large amounts of poly-unsaturated fat. They eventually went to Minnesota to run further studies on the Eskimo blood in the laboratory of Dr. Mark Holman, the world's fat expert at that time.

He found the Eskimos had a high concentration of the good cholesterol, HDL, the one that cleans out your arteries, low levels of bad cholesterol LDL, and even lower levels of very low-density LDL or bad cholesterol. Gas chromatography was needed to differentiate the different fats. What I'm saying is that all fat is not the same. Essential fatty acids, unsaturated fats and some poly-unsaturated fats can be good for you; saturated, or hydrogenated, fats are killers. They were separated apart by their boiling points and molecular weight.

The omegas got their name from Dr. Mark Holman.

It's my opinion the reason the Eskimos didn't develop these chronic diseases is related to the critical essential fatty acids they were consuming as well as their low consumption of the evil twin, fructose, and its malignant brother, glucose.

Dr. Holman wrote in 1964, "The concept of a balanced diet must include a ratio of several essential fat asses including mono-unsaturated, unsaturated, Omega-3's etc." The U.S. Department of Agriculture doesn't mention that in the most recent dietary recommendations. Fat was vilified in the 1960s, vegetable oil was vilified in the 1980s, trans fats in the 1990s and look at the result. The public is so confused that they still don't know what they should take most of the time, and, if they do, they don't know why they're taking it.

Dr. Ralph Holman has studied fats most of his professional life. Interestingly enough Dr. Ancel Keys, the enemy of fat, was also from Minnesota. He had a strong personality and few were willing to question his theory. But then again this was before a lot of the different fats were understood, according to a lot of scientists, although he never adjusted his opinion after new information become available.

The point is that all fats are not alike.

People had less heart disease during and after World War II and they were eating less meat, butter, cheese, and eggs. That has been well studied. When the above foods returned, people got sick again. Dr. Bang and Dr. Dyerberg did not know that they had upset the old model of Ancel Keys.

The omega-6s, which are pro-inflammatory, promote blood clotting, vasoconstriction, pain, cell division, depression, decreased effectiveness of the immune system and increased memory loss.

So now we know some of the history of essential fatty acids. As a reminder, they should be in a proper ratio of 1 to 1, 2 to 2 or 3 to 2, not 20 to 1.

In 2005, the Studer Group studied 275,000 subjects. In the study, omega-3s were shown to reduce risk factors by 32% and mortality by 23%. That is a huge statistic. What you eat and drink has a tremendous effect on your health.

More than 70 clinical trials have demonstrated the consistent glycemic lowering effect of fish oil supplements. Some studies have shown a triglyceride reducing effect as high as 79% compared to controls. Dr. Joe C. Maroon's book "Fish Oil" describes this in detail.

The main cause of vascular disease is inflammation. We have 300,000 miles of microvasculature, which is pretty amazing when you think about it. Vascular disease is the main cause of death globally, although cancer may surpass that statistic this year.

The main cause of vascular disease is turning on the fat switch; it's the twin's glucose and fructose, especially the latter – it's not cholesterol and some fats are even good.

The infiltration of our organs, including the liver, pancreas, and even our heart, by fat produced by the metabolism of fructose is the real Lex Luther, according to Dr. Robert Lustig.

All of this causes inflammation throughout our body, which means many people throughout the world are on fire. You don't see the flames because they are hidden in their body, but the results will show up sometime, in some very quickly.

When getting your blood work done, it is important to differentiate between LDL and VLDL. The very low-density LDL has such small molecules it takes a special test to diagnose them; one test is called "NMR" test and is not ordered routinely, so you have to ask for it. That is very important, since your life is at stake.

How do you put omega-3s back into your diet?

1) Consume oils that have a healthy balance of omega-3's and omega-6. Consume more flaxseed, walnuts, canola and soybean oils. Olive oil is good but limit it to 1 tablespoon daily, since, after all, it's 100% fat.

2) Eat lots of fruits and vegetables. Remember all plants contain some alpha-linoleic acid, the good fat.

3) Eat ocean-raised fish. Most fish today is raised on a farm and should be avoided. It is full of omega-6x versus ocean fish, which has many omega-3s.

4) Include some source of omega-3 in every meal. Add some nuts to your salads and you'll be doing it.

5) Avoid hydrogenated oils. They are full of trans fats and are not good for you.

6) Choose free-range chicken. Avoid animal products from organized farming organizations. They eat bad fats and you in turn will eat a lot of omega-6s. Likewise, when fish are fed corn.

7) Cut down on saturated fats. Fats are not as much a concern as fructose but if you're overweight, they will become a problem.

8) Check your BMI and maintain a healthy weight. I encourage you to weigh yourself every day, make a mental picture of what you want like to look at in 3 months and celebrate small losses.

CHO-Carbohydrate Metabolism

A CARBOHYDRATE IS A COMPLEX sugar compound and has to be broken apart to be metabolized. Some compounds have a lot of fiber, especially resisted starch. About 25% of the calories may be lost in metabolism because of the fiber and that's the good news. So it's not calories in and calories out.

But when carbohydrates are metabolized, the part that is absorbed is glucose and fructose. And they are used up, stored or changed to fat.

In 1750, we consumed 4 pounds of sugar yearly, in 1850, 20 pounds yearly, in 1994, 120 pounds, in 1990, it was 160 pounds. Let's face it, now it's probably around 200 pounds. This is well described by Nora T. Gedgaudas in "Primal Body, Primal Mind."

This estimate does not include all the hidden sources of sugar found in our thousands of manufactured foods. This doesn't even count high fructose corn syrup, which has been estimated to be about 80 pounds per year in the American diet. This huge increase can cause severe metabolic damage to us.

Our bodies are revolting in response to this onslaught on our genetic history.

Under the statistics, include the amount of sugar in our diets from other sources like carbohydrates, starches, cereals, breads, pastas, grains, potatoes and other types of sugar.

This is insanity.

Fruit, more than 2-3 pieces unfortunately is not a health food either, as fructose is the main sugar and is different from the fruits of millions of years ago. They have been seriously genetically modified to be sweeter as that is what sells. The industry knows the limits of our sweet tooth. Sugar sells, the sweeter it is the better it sells.

Sugar is both a carbohydrate and eventually a fat. That is what Dr. Robert Lustig emphasizes. The sugar stimulates an increase in insulin. Which is an anabolic hormone and causes weight increase.

Sugar and carbohydrates stimulate insulin, the anabolic fat storage hormone, which by process of glycation combines protein and sugar forming advanced glycation end product, AGEs, which are the cause of a lot of diseases.

Bread, pastas, cereals, potatoes, fried food, desserts, alcohol and unfortunately much of the fruit we eat have a great deal of fructose and you must be aware of that.

We accept blood glucose levels of 85-100, but our ancestors were averaging probably 70-85 levels.

Longevity studies are revealing 70-85 is a lot healthier if you don't develop hypoglycemia. We are not used to those levels so that might happen. Our ancestors probably had no problem with that.

The rule of thumb is that the lower your HBA 1C is, the longer you will live. It's a marker of aging.

The less sugar you eat, the better will be your health. A bagel contains 6 teaspoons full of glucose, I admit I ate a dozen once after a stressful day. Remember the fructose will not turn your appetite off like glucose might.

Cereals and potatoes can raise blood sugar levels faster than a candy bar.

Glucose in the bloodstream, especially fructose, oxidize and release free radicals, creating advanced glycation end products (AGEs) and secondary inflammation throughout the body.

Keytones from fats are more stable and don't raise the blood sugar or insulin level and can supply fuel for the brain. They also cause bad breath. Our red blood cells need oxygen and sugar to function in all the stages of our life. They create the energy molecule ATP.

Aging is now being understood by people who research longevity as essentially a gradual process of glycation. Chronic disease is associated with aging and certain forms of dementia. You see a lot more dementia in type II diabetics.

Whenever glucose is not immediately used for the acute activities of life, physical activity for example, and maintaining the metabolism of our body, is converted to glycogen. This stored glycogen in the liver and muscles will be converted to fat.

Glucagon, epinephrine, norepinephrine, cortisone and growth hormone also regulate blood sugar. Blood sugar lowering is a trivial sideline for insulin, contrary to what most people know about it.

Nature never would've made us totally dependent on just one mechanism of blood sugar control, it's too important.

We need a steady flow of fuel. Our bodies with our consumption of fructose are basically on fire. We need to feed directly, consistently and that's why we are creating the fuel. We have adapted our bodies to do this.

Contrary to most knowledge, alcoholics have issues with sugar addiction. Alcoholics are dependent and seek out fast sources of sugar, like alcohol, which is rapidly absorbed and metabolized in the liver, unfortunately, some of it goes to the brain. Once an alcoholic, always an alcoholic. It's a quick sugar fix. We need to eat daily.

I know a couple people who had a problem with alcohol, but only gained a little bit of weight, largely because of poor nutrition and lack of exercise; once they stopped consuming alcohol, they gained a lot of weight. They exploded with their sugar addiction. I'm concerned about their livers. First alcohol and its sugars causing fatty liver and now all the fructose through the consumption of sugary foods is doing a double whammy to their liver.

The real problem is addiction to glucose and fructose.

Go to any AA meeting and what are they serving? Doughnuts and cookies, which serve to further feed the addiction.

Nora T. Gedgaudas calls them "carbovores." I call them respectfully "carboholics."

Turning the body more in the direction of low sugar and good fats is the answer.

Nature would never have held us only dependent on sugar.

Our primal ancestors would never have made it only on a sugar diet.

Most people adapted to a state of carbohydrate and sugar metabolism and look at the result-obesity and chronic disease. Most people manage their blood sugar levels by eating sugary foods all day long.

They need to stoke the fire that's occurring in their body.

Dietary fat, in the absence of carbohydrate, is like putting a nice big log on the fire. It keeps going for long time and reduces the ups and downs. Fat does not raise blood sugar quickly and only when it's used up in energy metabolism.

Metabolically we are having a failure to communicate with our evolutionary hormonal system. Only one percent of the pancreas is devoted to insulin secretion.

Type II diabetes is a disease of the blood sugar because of insulin resistance. That's why the level of insulin in the blood is more important even than the blood sugar level, especially in the 10 to 15 years before a diagnosis is ever made. A recent study published in the "New England Journal of Medicine 2008" stated that they were surprised to find that increased insulin use actually caused an increase in death from heart attack and stroke. It was the result of the ACCORD study. The study was actually cut short due to these alarming findings. This unfortunately continues to be the standard in diabetic care, a focus on blood sugar instead of insulin resistance. The key is the restoration of insulin sensitivity and cellular communication.

The great fire: atherosclerosis

CARDIOLOGIST FOR MANY DECADES HAVE promoted the idea that atherosclerosis affects the larger blood vessels and is caused by cholesterol and fat in the diet. It was promoted as the "fat theory of vascular disease." As it turns out it's mainly the sugar, glucose and fructose, the omega-6's from vegetable oils and non-organic animal and fish farming. The latter cause a low-grade inflammatory process throughout the body. Inflammatory chemicals are attacking the surface of the blood vessels, trying to gobble up the very low density LDL and triglycerides and starting the process of arteriosclerosis and atherosclerosis. If enough of these inflammatory cells form, they become both visible and dangerous, something I've seen many times as a neurosurgeon.

Increasing evidence indicates that atherosclerosis is an inflammatory disease; that theory has been buttressed by studies that show that the predictive power of a marker of inflammation called C-reactive protein, CRP, increases with increasing atherosclerosis and arteriosclerosis. Your CRP should be less than one, a relative of mine was tested recently at 13, her whole side of the family has type II diabetes; I suspect she has vascular disease unfortunately.

Inflammatory events cause the liver to make CRP. It can raise very high levels if inflammation and is occurring throughout the body.

CRP was discovered 70 years ago, and cardiologists found CRP to be a predictor of future heart attacks or strokes. CRP, very low density LDL and HbA1c are good health screening tests.

The chemical insulin has been found to cause inflammation and diabetes is an inflammatory disease. Insulin resistance is phase 1 of development of diabetes. Some people call it diabesity at that stage. Probably 100,000,000 to 150,000,000 people have that in this country if they were properly tested. Because of vascular inflammation, type II diabetics essentially all have hypertension and vascular disease. If you have type II diabetes you have vascular disease. So prevention is the key.

Overweight individuals have increased levels of fatty acids-especially omega-6's which cause insulin resistance. Americans run a very high rate of omega-6's in the body that cause inflammation. The average American consumes a 20-1 omega-6 to omega-3 ratio. It should be more like one-to-one. The more we are like metabos (overweight), the more inflammatory fat cells we make in the inflammatory cells that cause insulin resistance, which over number years turns into type II diabetes. Most likely our bodies have been on fire for decades and we just didn't see it. Good laboratory testing would have revealed it and given us the chance to turn things around. It's never too late.

The Real Enemy

THE REAL ENEMY IN TYPE 2 diabetes is insulin resistance. Our body requires energy: ATP, adenosine triphosphate. It's a gasoline to run the machinery of our body. Some cells, muscles and neurons require a lot more energy than others. Sugar provides energy that comes from food, usually carbohydrates.

Food starts breaking down with the chemicals and saliva in your mouth with its enzymes. Enzymes and acids break it down further in the stomach and intestines and eventually it ends up as sugar and enters the bloodstream. Now the pancreas gets to work and figures out the level of energy needed in the body and secretes insulin. It secretes insulin according to what the level of blood sugar is. Its job is to open the door of the cell to let in the sugar that can be converted with oxygen to the energy molecule ATP. It locks onto receptors on the surface of the cell, of which there are thousands on every cell, and sends a message to the inside of the cell to open the door to let the sugar in. A messenger from inside the cells says open the door to sugar.

Insulin is a chemical messenger. It signals proteins called Glut-4 transporters, which rise to the cell membrane, where they grab onto glucose and take it inside.

Insulin resistance occurs because fat makes your receptors sticky and insulin can't knock on the door of the cell.

The pancreas responds by sending out more insulin, more door knockers, sometimes to an excessive amount. Sugar eventually makes its way into the cell, but because the insulin level remains high in the blood, which is very damaging to the body, this can lead to inflammation, arteriosclerosis, and many other effects throughout the body. Insulin resistance is the first step in the development of type 2 diabetes. This explains why type 2 diabetics all have insulin resistance.

Over time, the pancreas wears out and the beta cells begin to die. Now we have type 1 diabetes also, which entails insulin shots. You don't make enough insulin now; you have to take it externally in addition to some oral medications.

Insulin resistance causes more trouble than diabetes, potentially leading to obesity, hypertension, high cholesterol, low-density cholesterol, strokes, heart attacks, and some forms of cancer. About 125 million people in the United States probably have metabolic syndrome and insulin resistance is the center of it.

Insulin resistance is in the crosshairs of syndrome X, a synonym for metabolic syndrome.

Over 90% of diabetics that I have met have no idea what causes it. Many are at fault in this situation: I think we medical providers need to take the majority of the blame. Then again all of us need to participate in our healthcare. Unfortunately, only about 50% of the diabetics are compliant with their provider. Who knows for sure where the fault lies, but let's face it and try to fix it. Incidentally, I've written a book "Motivating to Wellness," which may help one make the necessary lifestyle changes.

About 75% of the people who have metabolic syndrome have no idea that they have it. Probably 25% have a fatty liver, a disease that is largely the cause of insulin resistance.

I generally make drawings for patients to teach them what insulin resistance is, see them back monthly if they wish, have them listen to CDs, have them watch DVDs that I've made and that seems to motivate them because they realize my heart is in it. Together, we all need to keep on trying.

One provider told me that the patients don't want to change. I think he's wrong and that and we just have to figure out what motivates each patient. Believe me, most people will eventually get the point and give it a shot. When you eat the right food, type 2 diabetes decreases or vanishes in about 60 days, 80 to 90% of the time. Dr. Franklin House wrote a book called "The 30 Day Miracle" and says he can do it in 30 days.

Dr. Raven from Stanford University has been the world leader in the study of insulin resistance. He discusses the relationship between insulin resistance, hypertension, obesity, high lipids, low-density LDL, metabolic syndrome, and insulin resistance syndrome, or syndrome X. About 50% of the people who have metabolic syndrome will develop type 2 diabetes. No one knows the exact percentage for sure.

When there is too much sugar circulating in the blood, it can clog up small blood vessels by several different methods. Sugar metabolism increases free radicals; sugar attaches to the proteins and can damage the blood vessels in the eyes, kidneys, brain and extremities, causing significant harm. When it comes to affecting the nerves, it can lead to diabetic neuropathy, a disease characterized by pain, numbness and weakness that can lead to loss of extremities including amputations. Symptoms will develop including burning, itching, numbness, pain and paralysis. The symptoms may be confused with spinal problems, ruptured disks and stenosis. The pain can be excruciating.

Much evidence indicates that there is a link between diabetes and hypertension and it is due to hyperinsulinemia. A state of cellular resistance to insulin action sets up the observed hyperinsulism. The reason for the association of insulin resistance and essential hypertension can be seen in at least 4 general types of mechanisms: sodium retention, sympathetic nervous system over-activity, disturbed membrane ion transport and perforation of vascular smooth muscle cells. Last, insulin, besides causing hypertension and obesity, is also known as atherogenic. It enhances cholesterol transport into arterial smooth muscle cells and increases endogenous lipid substances by the cells. Insulin stimulates production of various blood vessel growth factors. Also, insulin resistance increases serum uric acid, which is a cause of hypertension.

In summary, insulin resistance appears to be a syndrome that is associated with the clustering of metabolic disorders, including non-insulin dependent diabetes, obesity, hypertension, cancer and atherosclerotic cardiovascular disease. These cytokines in abdominal and liver fat lead to insulin resistance. Probably 25% of Americans have non-alcoholic fatty liver disease and the majority of them don't know it.

About 20 to 30% of normal weight individuals have insulin resistance and metabolic syndrome. So if BMI is not the last word, CRP, liver function tests, MRI or ultrasound, homocysteine, lipid profile, especially low-density LDL, a 2-hour glucose tolerance test which includes blood sugar are all important for diagnosis.

Millions of years ago, living things, fish, amoeba, protozoa, microbes, communicated from cell to cell with eicosanoids, one-cell fatty acids. There was no blood system and we still have that communicating system in our body today.

When you get a paper cut, prostaglandins respond and cause redness and pain and the leukotrines command and produce the chemicals of inflammation. They direct your white cell army of Marines and Navy.

Obesity is now considered an inflammatory disease because insulin resistance is an inflammatory process. It is caused by the fat, salt and sugar that we eat on a daily basis as well as smoking. At age 60, half of the people in the United States have at least one chronic disease: severe arthritis, heart disease, strokes, dementia, Parkinson's disease, and 100 million people with pre- and type 2 diabetes heading towards 150 million people.

The devil of the inflammatory story is AA, arachidonic acid. It makes the prostaglandins and leukotriene's.

It was discovered in the late 1800s that aspirin could block the inflammatory response by inhibiting that Cox one enzyme. It resulted in the Bayer aspirin, which helped a lot of people by stopping a lot of the inflammatory response in its tracks.

Can we stop inflammation before it starts? It turns out that aspirin stops the prostaglandin pathway but not the leukotriene pathway. It can help the problem but it can't cure it.

The problem is we get a great deal of AA in our Western diets. Farm-raised fish for example versus ocean fish. Dietary AA and heart disease, diabetes, cancer etc. have been connected in scientific studies.

Older people have increased levels of AA, which is part of the aging process; we are, indeed, rusting.

Some government supported super foods are actually making us sick! Let's look at salmon, for example. Great health food because of anti-inflammatories Omega 3s? Wrong. 90 percent of our salmon today comes from a feedlot and not the ocean, fed by government supported fat and sugar.

Farm-fed salmon is full of AA, the pro-inflammatory chemical. Ocean fish live on algae, plants, sardines and not soybean products, carbon products, chicken litter as they have on aqua farms. Always ask your waiter where their fish came from, the ocean or feedlot. We can indeed change things if we do that enough.

Ocean salmon is full of EPA and DHA, the good eicosanoids. Remember these are the terms you want to remember for good supplements. A 4-ounce farm-raised salmon can have up to 1,300 grams of AA. This has been scientifically studied. If you need scientific proof read the book called "Inflammation Nation" by Dr. Floyd H. Chilton, Ph.D.

2 fried eggs have 146 mg of AA and should be avoided. So poach your eggs and avoid frying. There are actually high levels of AA in lean turkey, and pork is even higher in AA.

So what is the anti-inflammatory diet?

Avoid animal meat, including farm-fed fish, and salt and sugar. Sugar is pro-inflammatory because it is a carbohydrate as well as a fat. The fructose in sugar is your real enemy because of its chemistry and metabolism. I recommend an 80% plant-based diet, with carefully selected lean meat. Get at least 30 minutes of exercise a day no matter what. You just have to commit to it until it gets to be a habit. I also do some tai chi while I'm walking; it's automatic and also is now a habit. Exercise helps the metabolism, and greatly improves the chemistry of your body while reducing stress. Most of us use sugar as a narcotic to relieve the stress. I wouldn't overdo it in supplements but I generally recommend some vitamin D, Omega-3 and a multivitamin and that's about it. Don't overdo it in supplements because they also have side effects. You're much better off eating 100% whole grain, if not gluten sensitive, vegetables, foods with fiber, little animal products and some fruit. I also wrote "The Secret of the Non-diet" for further information.

Inflammation

OUR HEALTH IS BEING DESTROYED by the effects of out-of-control inflammation.

It's the toxic food we're eating and drinking.

The epidemic of inflammation is a bigger cause of disease then our genetic structure. The government is putting the majority of research money into gene research. But it's what we were eating and drinking that causes majority of our illnesses, yet we are devoting very few healthcare dollars to study that.

Being overweight, having metabolic syndrome and type 2 diabetes is the consequence of increasing insulin resistance in the blood. The cause of type 2 diabetes, which is all around us, are inflammation and insulin resistance.

Inflammation is the monkey on your back, and the predecessor of insulin resistance. If there were no inflammation, you wouldn't have insulin resistance, and the resultant diseases and illnesses brought on by that.

Dr. Mehmet Oz says, "Inflammation is the rusting of your arteries." Inflammation is a fire where you can't see the flames.

It remains hidden for many years until you run some tests, and then it might be too late.

The immune system involves your thymus, spleen, bone marrow, white blood cells —they are your Army, Navy, Air Force and Marines, which are supposed to win the war and bring you back to good health. This happens when you may have a local infection. But in your body it's an unending war, with your arteries and nerves involved with chronic infection because we continue to supply the body with toxic foods like salt and sugar. As Dr. Herbert Benson from Harvard would say, there is a doctor living within everyone's body, the immune system that knows how to repair things. We are attempting to repair the chronic inflammation but are causing a lot of damage in the process.

Your low density LDL infiltrates the interior walls of you arteries and capillaries; the inflammatory process with its macrophages jumps in to try to repair the problem and causes plaque formation instead. This causes arterial narrowing and can lead to trouble. The inflammatory process occurs throughout the body, and in the brain it can lead to dementia.

Eventually inflammation leads to vascular disease, strokes, heart attacks, glaucoma, arthritis, kidney disease, neuropathy etc., and it can inflame your 300,000 miles of capillary blood vessels.

The realization that the immune system plays a role in the onset of most major diseases has now been well proven. The immune system is a major killer stimulated by what we eat and what we do.

One million teenagers have metabolic syndrome based on inflammation. This speaks poorly of the future. Inflammation destroys the body by friendly fire. We are destroying our bodies by what we do or don't do. We're shooting ourselves in the head on a daily basis. Just look around you: Most people are totally unaware of what they are doing to themselves or they're just closing their eyes.

Our nation is dying from bad food. Oxidation is the process of aging. It's like trying new food with a decaying fruit like a banana. It makes your apple brown and its skin wrinkles. This is the aging process. Smoking is a cause of inflammation and we all know that smokers may look 20 years older than they really are.

Macrophages are powerful immune cells that are sent into the arterial walls and can cause thrombosis and in turn a heart attack.

Anything that causes inflammation will in turn cause insulin resistance, and anything that causes insulin resistance will cause inflammation. They are the evil twins.

We can easily identify inflammation from a sore throat, which is obvious, but the inflammation in our body can be hidden and turn into diseases and illnesses, resulting in chronic disease, disability and death.

The inflammation that drives obesity and chronic disease is invisible and doesn't hurt. It's a hidden smoldering fire created by **your immune system** that is trying to fight off bad food, sugar, fat and salt in processed food as well as smoking.

What triggers the inflammatory process?

Sugar is number one, refined carbohydrates, trans fats and too many Omega-6s from animal meets and plant oils. Also artificial sweeteners, high fructose corn syrup, food sensitivities, gut bacteria, genetic makeup, food additives and chemicals, meat produced by concentrated animal feeding organizations, fish grown in feedlots, as well as gluten.

Mounting evidence underscores the critical role that inflammation plays in the development of type 2 diabetes.

Dietary sugars and refined flours are the biggest triggers of inflammation. They cause insulin levels to spike and start a cascade of biochemical reactions that turn on our gene's chronic inflammation.

Lack of fiber, too many inflammatory Omega-6s and not enough Omega-3s, plus anti-inflammatory essential fats lead to the development of systemic inflammation throughout the body.

Food sensitivities and allergies also add to the problem. Many people have gluten sensitivity and not a true allergy but they get sick anyhow with many systemic type symptoms but it is not as deadly, unless they have celiac disease.

Many of the reactions and allergies are from a "leaky gut" created by proteins, byproducts of food digestion that leak through holes in the gut. This occurs much more commonly with the reaction to genetically modified new foods. They have no evolutionary history. Many foods have been genetically modified. Our bread is not what it used to be; it's more of a Franken food, a byproduct of industrial agriculture.

The Story of Fat

FAT IS A TRIGLYCERIDE. 3 fatty acid molecules and one glycerol molecule

- Not all fat is bad; we need to eat some **essential fatty acids** every day because they are not made by our body. Most of us have heard the term Omega-3 and Omega-6 and these are the important essential fatty acids that we need. Omega-3 fatty acids, found in wild fish, are anti-inflammatory.
- Monounsaturated fats include olive and canola oil
- Some Unsaturated fats such as omega-3's are anti-inflammatory
- Saturated fatty acids – non-grass fed animal meat, milk and dairy products – cause atherosclerosis
- Medium chain triglycerides – palm oil, coconut oil – are a good energy source, with some suggestion of atherosclerosis
- Omega-6 fatty acids – from farm raised animals and fish and some vegetable oils – can cause atherosclerosis, insulin resistance, and immune dysfunction, are pro-inflammatory.

Before living things developed a circulatory system, single cell essential fatty acids jumped from cell to cell and those are the omega-3 and omega-6 fatty acids. They are anti-inflammatory, and they are the communicating systems between 70 trillion cells, so you can see how important they are. Without them we would not exist. The good eicosanoids prevent blood clots, cause vasodilatation, reduce pain, reduce cell division, enhance immunity and improve brain function.

The bad eicosanoids, the Omega-6's, promote blood clotting, cause vasoconstriction, promote pain, promote cell division, depress the immune system, cause inflammation and mental depression.

So Omega-3s are anti-inflammatory and sources are fish oil, flaxseed, nuts and vegetables.

The good Omega-3s include ALA, EPA and DHA. Omega-6s include LA, AAA, GLA and DGLA.

The 4 foods of the apocalypse are trans fats, alcohol, fructose and branch-chained amino acids.

Metabos

THE JAPANESE A FEW YEARS ago had a national vote to see if they could come up with a word that was friendlier than obesity.

Yes, they had a national vote and decided on Metabos.

Being a "metabo," you're more likely to develop a chronic disease like heart disease, stroke, vascular disease, Alzheimer's disease, cancer and autoimmune disease.

What comes first: obesity, diabetes, or inflammation?

Being a metabo comes first. The wheat belly actually is very dangerous. What we are eating today was genetically changed in 1948 at the Rockefeller Institute outside Mexico City. They increased the yield 10 times. The amylopectin in wheat heads straight for the liver and causes inflammation. Unfortunately fat sitting on your belly is in the liver, heart, and pancreas and generally not under the skin. It's a great cause of inflammation. Fat is very active metabolically. Metabolism is the sum activity of the chemical reactions in your body. It doesn't just sit there. Fat cells are micro-factories, a large amount of the chemical reactions that affect the body occur there. It's not just the liver. Fat cells act as a control center for many of the processes that determine how our body behaves.

Metabos have a chronic inflammatory disease. I see the body on fire when I visualize a metabo. Remember, this is a judgment-free zone.

What does the hibernating animal do? It stores fat, but it has a fat switch in the spring and they burn off their fat very quickly. Very few animals are fat unless fed by humans. They may be temporarily so to survive but not in the long run.

Overweight people have bigger fat cells, they can increase the storage 1,000 times. Generally, though, humans do not grow more fat cells.

Obese people make more of everything except adiponectin. The latter chemical is anti-inflammatory but it's decreased in the overweight population. This increases the formation of pro-inflammatory chemicals and decreases TNF, an anti-inflammatory.

The good and the bad: fat

WE KNOW NOW THAT WE have to take in some essential fatty acids because we do not make them and they are needed for our health. Our body would not work without them; they are our Intel chips of our body, they jump from cell to cell. Our 70 trillion body cells are totally dependent on them. They are in the cell membranes, cholesterol and omega-3's and omega-6's are essential to our life. The omega-3's are also called alpha-linolenic acid, the good guys. The omega-6's also called linolenic acid and are the pro-inflammatory. We need some of both but not in the proportion that we are eating them. So you can see we have good and bad essential fatty acids. AA also called arachidonic acid is pro-inflammatory.

In the 1980s all fats were considered bad. The American Heart Association put their labels on low-fat foods and made significant money from it. Essentially giving us that advice and getting paid for it. A wave of low-fat foods hit the grocery market.

In the 1990s they recommended different types of fats, vegetable oils, hydrogenated oils. Eventually these were found they made us sick too. Olive oil and omega-3's were recommended, the monounsaturated oils had more omega-3's in them. If you're trying to lose weight, remember though that all vegetable oils are 100% fat.

We now know that all unsaturated fats are not the same.

The polyunsaturated fats can be divided as already mentioned largely into 2 groups, omega-3, like in fatty fish or olive oil, and omega-6's like in soybean oil and non-organic meat.

Our body cannot make them so they are called essential fatty acids and without them we would risk heart disease, strokes cancer and numerous other illnesses. Healthy people, especially vegetarians, consume very few omega-6's. We Americans actually eat a huge amount of omega-6 in our Western diet. We are eating a pro-inflammatory diet--no wonder we're sick.

Saturated fats

IT WAS NATURAL FOR PEOPLE to switch to olive oil cooking to get away from saturated fats, because of the low-fat craze. However, olive oil is more expensive than the other polyunsaturated vegetable oils.

Replacing saturated fats such as lard, suet, and tallow, which are solid at room temperature, was a challenge. The only way to do that was through a process called hydrogenation. This process led to the growth and mass production of fast food. Crisco and entirely new animal fat substitutes entered the market in 1911. Margarine and Crisco were both top sellers in the first half of the 20th century.

It took nearly 2 decades for these trans fats to be recognized by the FDA as questionable for human health. How did this happen? Vegetable oil produces influenced the scientific research on trans fats. High-level tactics are routinely employed by the large oil companies.

After 50 years of promoting the low-fat diet by the American Heart Association, NIH, the government along with Ancel Keys and Associates finally came out and said that fat theory is in the process of being defeated. Hydrogenated vegetable oils were then promoted.

The Center for Science in the Public Interest, based in Washington D.C., is a very powerful and focused consumer group.

The CSPI urged fast food companies such as Burger King, McDonald's and others to abandon beef tallow (fat) for partially hydrogenated oil. A major error. This was done especially in frying French fries. Saturated fats were replaced with "healthy hydrogenated oils."

All the major food companies removed the fat and replaced it with vegetable oils. This was done due to the CSPI claim.

Retailers were urged to switch to hydrogenated oils or popcorn, from butter and coconut oil to hydrogenated oils. This created a huge industry. They were dead wrong.

Another force pushing the food companies to stop using saturated fats was a multimillionaire in Nebraska named Phil Sokolov, according to reporter Nina Teicholz who wrote the great book "The Big Fat Surprise." His main target was coconut and palm oils. They were largely made in foreign countries and U.S. vegetable oil companies had been fighting their importation for decades. He said that palm oil has 25% more saturated fat than lard and that coconut oil has 5% more than lard.

He placed many national ads and tried to influence the American diet big time. The American Soybean Association also ran a big anti-saturated fat campaign. Politics and company money were at play.

Lobbying by the industry killed the palm oil and coconut oil industry in this country. It was the soybean industry at work.

These campaigns, for example, said that 70% of soybean oil is hydrogenated. The U.S. population knew very little about hydrogenation and its effects. Ultimately the American Soybean Association backed down because it was offered a deal by the Asian Palm and Coconut Oil Association.

That ended a 2-year feud. Trans fats were now used everywhere. This produced a national disaster, the fast food industry grew in leaps and bounds. We ate 18,000,000 pounds of soybean oil in 2001.

Truth about trans-fats

IN THE 1920S AND '30S, many people were ambivalent about fats and trans fats as the cause of disease.

A 1944 study, however, established a perception that trans fats were okay. And then hydrogenated oils flooded the food supply for the next 40 years. The study was done by Best Foods, the manufacturer of margarine, and done on rats. They gave trans fats a clear bill of health.

In 1961 Ancel Keys turned his attention to trans fats. He found that hydrogenated oils increased total cholesterol; they also were shown to increase LDL and increased triglycerides.

Procter & Gamble, brought Crisco to the market in 1911, which is full of trans fat. We're talking money here.

Over the next 20 years, a Dr. Kumerow, a professor of biochemistry at the University of Illinois, produced more than 70 scientific papers on trans fats during the course of his career.

The first study was published in Science magazine in 1957. He examined autopsy material for 24 subjects and actually found trans-fats had a cumulative pall over their bodies, liver, arteries, and especially in the fat. He thought that they were not properly metabolized. Also, a lot of these trans fats had become calcified and the body was unable to remove them. The latter is the reason we now do CT scans of the heart and calculate our calcium scores, which is very important and very interesting.

Dr. Kumerow was a political innocent. The American Heart Association received millions from the food industry. Kumerow even criticized the American Heart Association medical director for posing with a bottle of Crisco.

Remember the American Heart Association was recommending the prudent diet that was low in saturated fat and high in vegetable oils in 1961. Liquid oil was eventually substituted for hydrogenated oil. Then the American Heart Association endorsed polyunsaturated oils even though they were aware of Dr. Kumerow's work.

Kumerow became persona non grata at the AHA.

Kumerow was met with a wall of silence. Over 40 years, few colleagues wanted to speak to him or even communicate with him.

The Difference between Type 1 and Type 2 Diabetes

TYPE 1 DIABETES IS WHERE you do not make enough insulin to push sugar into the cells for energy. It was considered a juvenile disease, but, it actuality can occur at any age. Some type 2 diabetics can eventually become type 1, and that is the majority of the patients.

Type 2 diabetes is due to insulin resistance and the inability of insulin to push sugar into the cell. 90 percent of diabetics are type 2, and 90% of them may develop type 1 because the pancreas just wears out secreting insulin at a high rate.

Glucose is a sugar and the largest source of energy in the body. Sugar and oxygen chemically react and produce adenosine-triphosphate (ATP) in the mitochondria, or work station, of our body's 70 trillion cells. Without this chemical reaction, we would not be alive. Each of our cells has at least 10,000 mitochondria.

It is very important that we maintain a normal blood sugar. A level too high or too low will have serious consequences. The hormone insulin, glucagon and the liver are all in charge of keeping the blood sugar within reasonable range. When the blood sugar is too low, the liver releases available stored sugar; the liver receives messages from insulin to increase or decrease the amount of sugar; and glucagon is available to stimulate sugar production or breakdown of glucagon, a form of sugar in the muscles and liver. If the system becomes overloaded, the liver will convert glucose or fructose into fat.

Glucagon is the opposite of insulin, and turns on the switch so that fatty acids can be used as an energy source, and it signals the body to increase sugar production.

Type 2 diabetes is preceded by a state of pre-diabetes or diabesity. The whole purpose of this book is to catch those patients at this stage before type 2 diabetes occurs. In pre-diabetes, insulin levels are elevated for many years, but blood sugars are normal, resulting in great damage to the body. A significant number of patients in the pre-diabetic state develop vascular disease, neuropathy, have heart attacks and strokes, increased rate of cancer, inflammatory disease of the blood vessels and nerves in the body.

10% of type 1 diabetes is usually diagnosed in childhood, but can occur at any age. It is considered an autoimmune disease, where the immune system attacks the pancreas; some cases are thought to be viral in origin.

Patients generally present with weight loss, tremendous thirst and hunger, lack of energy, and episodes of sweating. Blood and urine tests for sugar should be done. Remember, type 2, can lead to type 1 because the pancreas is sick and tired of secreting high amounts of insulin and just plain wears out.

There are other types of diabetes, for example gestational diabetes during pregnancy; a significant number (50%) of these patients go on to have type 2 diabetes in the future. Most of these women are pre-diabetic and the metabolic changes of pregnancy speed things up.

Any pancreatic damage, of course, could cause type 1 diabetes and autoimmune diseases, viral infections, bacterial infections, cancer, and mineral deposits like iron or calcium.

90 percent of type 2 diabetics can be prevented, stopped or reversed the majority of the time. Dr. Franklin House from Arizona thinks he can do it in 30 days, some as quickly as a week. Dr. Mark Hyman says it can be done in a week according to a heart study, It's strictly dependent on the type of food you're eating and we'll discuss that in more detail later. Most people have been pre-diabetic for 5 to 15 years before a clear diagnosis is made, which is a very sad situation because the body has already been damaged. This can lead to heart disease and heart attacks, ovarian or uterine cancer, nerve damage or kidney damage. A significant number have impaired vision.

"Early diagnosis" with a 2-hour glucose tolerance test is critical; this is essential, otherwise, you can miss the opportunity to avoid the disease altogether. Additional tests of course are important, including the usual fasting blood sugar, HbA1c, C. reactive protein, homocysteine and lipid profile. The correct diagnosis is critical. Testing may need to be repeated for clear diagnosis!

Today I had my hair cut by a young girl at Sweetwater, the great music distribution center where I was trying to arrange a music lesson. Her dad had a stroke at age 50. She's on her way to 180 pounds, with high blood pressure, and she's trying to tell me she's not type 2 diabetic or pre-diabetic. I bet that a provider never checked her insulin level with a 2-hour glucose tolerance test. I just know the story too well. I gave her names of books to read as this association can be stopped and possibly reversed. Dr. Dean Ornish proved it in his famous books, as well as Dr. Caldwell Esselstyn.

In summary type 2 diabetes is preceded by a pre-diabetic state where we have a "Golden Opportunity" to stop, prevent and reverse the situation.

Some divide type 2 diabetes into 5 stages:
- Stage 1 - insulin resistance (IR) only
- Stage 2 - IR, plus hyperinsulinism (HI)
- Stage 3 - IR, HI, plus abnormalities in a GTT
- Stage 4 - Type 2 diabetes, with high insulin levels
- Stage 5 - Type 2 diabetes, with low insulin levels, the end stage

Do you see the problem? If you're diagnosed with stage 5 there are serious consequences.

The disease is prevalent throughout our population and is a great threat to our health and well-being. This is a war worse than anything else attacking our country.

Our evolutionary bodies are not accustomed to what we are eating. We are eating 90% genetically altered, chemically altered, products of fat, salt and sugar and highly processed foods. Our evolutionary history only changes 0.2% every 20,000 years. We greatly changed our food source 10,000 years ago and then through the Industrial Revolution, chemical farming and government support of bad food, all of this is leading to what some people call the United States of Diabesity.

Big food fights back

THOMAS APPLEWHITE, THE ORGANIC PLANT physiologist and director of Kraft research, was unquestionably the leader of trans fat promotion, according to Nina Teicholtz's "The Big Fat Surprise."

Whenever Kumerow, who I mentioned in the previous chapter, spoke at a conference, he was literally attacked by other speakers, many of them representing the food industry. Applewhite was particularly intimidating because he was a tall individual. The industry knew that trans fats were linked to heart disease – the jig was up. Kumerow never gave up. In 2013, at age 93, he continued publishing papers. He was constantly pressuring the FDA to ban trans fat from the food supply altogether.

In a hostile environment that denies richer scientific research and discussion, ideas tend to die, especially if the research money is not forthcoming.

The beginning of the end of trans fat recommendations began in Europe with studies done by Martyn B Katau, a molecular biologist. The big European food company called Unilever financed his studies. We must give them credit for that. The results of the studies indicated that hydrogenated oils decreased the good HDL and increased the bad LDL, and when the hydrogenated oil is removed the results went the other way.

The end of trans fats

DR. WILLARD FROM HARVARD, WHO was the director of the Nurse's Health Study involving 100,000 nurses, studied cholesterol levels in women for many years.

He did make a couple of recommendations, which are eventually proving to be wrong. He recommended, for instance, that women take hormones after menopause and vitamin E, which have both since turned out to be incorrect.

He said, "Trans fats are a metabolic poison." Trans fats became the number one poison. In 2003 the FDA ruled that trans fat causes heart disease. The day that ruling came out, we had 43,000 foods with trans-fats in them.

They had to be removed from the frying of French fries at fast food restaurants and other foods.

Toxic heated vegetable oils

ANCEL KEYS, THE NIH, NHBLI and the USDA said fats are bad for us and cause heart disease. When they finally decided that was poor advice, they said trans fats and hydrogenated vegetable oils were better for us. But you'll soon read that they may actually be worse when used in a frying and fast food preparations.

We ready saw that Dr. Willis from Harvard came out against the trans fats from reviewing other studies.

In 2003 an international team concluded that Dr. Willard's annual questionnaire to the 100,000 nurses in his study was not of much use, because of the multiple criteria and lack of control.

Dr. Willett had a close relationship with the New England Journal of Medicine, which was published in his hometown of Boston.

He was able to publish a lot of papers because of the multiple varieties of questions he was asking and evaluating from the questionnaire answered by the 100,000 nurses, resulting in a lot of articles and influence.

Trans fats became the "phantom fat"

WHAT TO DO NOW? THE industry asked. Hard fats are essential to the industry.

Studies have indicated that vegetable oils increase cancer rates and have been of great concern.

A large body of research has demonstrated that vegetable oils increase omega-6 essential fatty acid, which competes with omega-3's, the anti-inflammatory commonly found in fish oil. Omega-3's and omega-6's are located in every one of our cell membranes and are extremely important for our survival. They are the primitive communicating system throughout our 70 trillion body cells. The tsunami of omega-6, the pro-inflammatory essential fatty acids that ended up body via vegetable oils, especially the ones that have been oxidized resulting in free radicals that cause aging and are destroying our body because of vascular disease. We are inflamed. This kind of inflammation causes cancer, heart disease and strokes.

Vegetable oils constitute 8% of all the calories Americans are consuming on average. Very few clinically significant trials on their function have been done.

The American Heart Association's most recent dietary review of vegetable oils was in 2009 and encouraged the public to eat more of them and to increase them to 5 to 10% of all calories.

We need a true 3-year clinical trial involving new omega-3s and 6's to establish for certain their metabolic significance.

A huge problem is heating vegetable oils, especially at fast food restaurants where it's done 24 hours a day over the country and the world.

McDonald's, Burger King, Wendy's and others replaced hydrogenated oils with regular vegetable oils. It is now known that heating vegetable oils raises toxic oxidation products, which results in free radicals that damage DNA in our body.

I saw an example of the danger of oxidized oils recently at a fast food restaurant that was being remodeled; I took a look at the drains and it was frightening.

According to Nina Teicholz, she called the Echo Lab company, whose responsibility it is to clear the pipes of all food restaurants, and they confirmed that damage to the drainage pipes and fast food restaurants. They also mentioned the fire damage from accidental fires where employee's shirts occasionally catch on fire.

Also increased cancer rates have been reported in fast food restaurant employees, according to a study in Britain and Sweden.

Olive oil, a mono saturated essential fatty acid has only one double bond to react with oxygen to cause oxidation so it is safer. Polyunsaturated oils have multiple double bonds of which vegetable oils except olive oil are an example. Interestingly enough, the saturated fats found in butter, lard, and coconut oil produced less free radicals than vegetable oils.

The Journal of Food Chemistry in 1999 said, "Warning, the family of polyunsaturated oils are damaging to your heart health." Do we need more information?

Most Americans don't realize that the nutritional advice is based on such a narrow set of health recommendations. Frankly, it's lack of knowledge that is killing us.

Our fat consumption has moved from saturated fats at the beginning of the 20th century to partially hydrogenated oils, or poly unsaturated oils, and we're sicker and more obese than ever. We're badly in need of leadership from the top.

We have been unwittingly subjugated to a chain of events starting with the elimination of animal fats, then exposing us to the aldehydes and formaldehyde of vegetable oils. The FDA may ban trans fats completely, which will make only unsaturated oils and oxidative products even more common.

We may be jumping from the frying plan into the fire; personally, I know we are already on fire. Our bodies are being inflamed by toxins such as glucose, poisonous fructose, oxidative free radicals including vegetable oils and meat that has not been raised in the ocean or on an organic farm.

The Low Sugar Way

LET'S FACE IT: CARBOHYDRATES ARE essentially broken down into glucose and fructose.

In 1863 in London a mortuary owner named William Banting published a "Letter on Corpulence." It sold more than 100,000 copies in France, Germany and Britain and the United States.

He himself had obesity problems with complaints of joint pain, hearing issues, bowel problems and more.

His doctor prescribed exercise, which he did but it didn't help him at all. This actually stimulated his appetite and decreased his energy.

An ENT specialist whom he was seeing with hearing problems recommended a low carbohydrate diet. He had noticed protruding ear canals as well as fat in the neck area, typical problems seen with sleep apnea.

He switched to 3 meals a day of meat, fish, or grain and avoided sugar and starchy foods. He also avoided milk, candy and starchy root vegetables. He lost 50 pounds and felt great, full of energy and his symptoms cleared up.

He died at age 81, far above the average age of mortality for Britain at that time.

Many physicians tried restricting total calories and that did not work.

We're now eating pro-inflammatory meat products. In other words there are good and bad fats now. Although high carbohydrate and sugar diets are even worse than the bad fats.

Elliott Dansworth at the University of Vermont found that eating too much of a **meat**-centered diet is nearly impossible, because your appetite will turn off. But most people could eat carbohydrates and sugar all day. Interesting!

We're looking at fat like an ATM machine, according to Nina Teicholtz.

The hormonal effects could explain the menopausal and puberty weight gain that females have.

We now know that insulin causes weight gain. It is an anabolic hormone resulting in obesity.

A person would lose weight, avoiding sugar and carbohydrates because of the absence of insulin. Fat does not cause increased insulin levels.

Then World War II appeared and the scientists went to war; the research was lost and then rediscovered.

In 1953 the New England Journal of Medicine published the famous review by Dr. Pennington.

Interestingly, that was the same year that Dr. Ancel Keys got started with his "fat theory" as the cause of heart disease.

Keys was better known and his theory prevailed. But I doubt he had read the great research by the French, German and English researchers. The quality of the research was different and quite good. Keys' information was based on population studies, not clinical or animal research controlled studies.

There was no experimental basis for his assumptions.

A Hungarian born obstetrician named Herman Taller practicing in New York, read Pennington's article and treated his patients with a low carb diet. He wrote a book called "Calories Don't Count."

Sugar and chronic disease

HOW DO SUGAR AND CARBOHYDRATES cause chronic diseases like heart disease, strokes, diabetes, cancer and autoimmune diseases?

In the mid-1800s they started seeing the Western diseases of hypertension, osteoarthritis, gallbladder disease and diabetes.

Everyone seemed to get better when sugar was replaced by fat. Mind you we're talking about the 1950s. So we've known for a long time that sugar and carbohydrates are the problem and not fat. This was ignored by Ancel Keys, the American Heart Association, the U.S. Department of Agriculture, the National Association of Heart, Lung, and Blood Institute, AMA, the Mcgovern commission and many other scientists. The American Heart Association was receiving a lot of money from Procter & Gamble, and in return they offered an endorsement with their heart label on fatty products like lard and Crisco.

That cancer might be caused by sugar and carbohydrates in modern diets was of concern to the doctors working with primitive populations. Cancer started appearing when they started eating the Western diet. From the Arctic to Africa, scientists followed the transition of ancient diets to Western diets of sugar and carbohydrates.

Whenever people started eating the Western diet, they developed heart disease, diabetes and cancer. This was an epidemic studied by many scientists.

A German doctor named Otto Schaefer visited the well-known Inuit tribe, studied by many scientists, in the Canadian Arctic in 1951. He was on Baffin Island where there was no Western food and a very low level of Western diseases.

The Hudson Bay Company began bringing in loads of Western food, including flour and molasses. Some communities ate this and others didn't get any of this type of food. This gave Otto an opportunity to study different cultures. The Inuit who ate the ancient way remained very healthy. The ones who ate the Western way became sick.

What was hard to understand was in spite of eating very few vegetables and having very little sunshine, they had no vitamin deficiencies including vitamin D, vitamin C and other multivitamins. That has been very difficult to explain.

He observed that the natives eating large amounts of sugar changed their health greatly over a 20-year period. Dr. Yudkin who wrote "White Sweet Deadly" claimed that a 20-year lag is typical of the time it takes for the Western chronic diseases to appear. I personally think that lag time is a lot shorter than that. In many people, 30 days of nothing but fast food could make someone diabetic.

Whenever the natives stopped eating meat, they replace it with sugar and carbohydrates. He told a local newspaper "it was self-inflicted genocide."

The British Royal Navy surgeon Capt. Thomas Cleve had seen some of the same phenomena in many remote areas to which he had been transferred in the early 1900s. He called the chronic disease "saccharine disease" and wrote a famous book later by that name. I highly recommend reading it. I wonder if Dr. Ancel Keys, American Heart Association, NIH, American Association of Heart and Lung Blood Institute ever read that book. Boatloads of sugar came to the British Isles in the 1670s. The slave trade was started over that. It didn't stop until the 1850s. People in Britain consumed about 4 pounds of sugar per year in 1670, which increased to 20 pounds in the 1800s and now is about 180 pounds a year like the United States – about a half a pound a day.

Heart disease began to appear in the mid-1800s, and it was thought that meant that sugar was the answer. Meat consumption stayed the same, but heart disease increased after that. The only element of the diet to keep pace with heart disease was sugar. Fat consumption stayed the same. Then Banting came along with his story and book. Rates of cancer also increased dramatically. Cancer went from being a rarity and was essentially unknown in the Eskimos and Indian tribes. We all know now cancer is a sugar feeder. 70 percent of uterine cancer occurs in overweight people, and about 30% of breast cancers are related to the estrogen in fat.

A Short Review

SUGAR MAY BE BAD, BUT the sweetener called fructose is far more deadly.

A 2009 study from the University of California, Davis, and additional scientific studies confirm that consuming high fructose corn syrup is the fastest way to trash your health. It is now known, without a doubt, that sugar in food, in all its myriad forms, is taking a devastating toll.

Fructose in any form, including high fructose corn syrup and crystalline fructose, is the worst of the worst. Fructose, a cheap sweetener usually derived from corn, is used in thousands of food products and soft drinks. Excessive fructose consumption can cause metabolic damage and trigger the early stages of diabetes and heart disease.

Dr. Richard Johnson does a fabulous job of comprehensively reviewing this important topic in his new book, "The Fat Switch." Fructose consumption leads to insulin resistance, obesity, elevated blood pressure, elevated triglycerides and elevated LDL, depletion of vitamins and minerals, cardiovascular disease, liver disease, fatty liver, cancer, arthritis and even gout.

Evil Twin Detox

IF YOU WANT TO RECLAIM your health, control your future, look and feel great, then I recommend standing in front of the mirror and visualizing what you want to look like in 6 months. Do it at least once a week. It can be motivating and stimulating. Create a plan and follow through.

Create a mantra, a few words that you say out loud at least twice a day that will motivate you. For example, "I want to get rid of my type 2 diabetes in 6 months," "I'm doing this for my family," "I want to look strong and fit."

To reduce the power of glucose and fructose, it is best to go through about 10 to 14 days of detox, a period where you are much stricter in your consumption of sugar, glucose and fructose than you normally need to be. I would even give up alcohol for 2 weeks because it is a sugar. This will reduce your fructose enzymes in the liver and stabilize the addictive power of sugar on the brain.

Nutrient-dense foods, through something called nutrigenomics, have acquired genes that affect food metabolism through epigenetics, in other words have the ability to repair your sick genes. Food is information. I was recently at a conference and an addiction specialist told me, you can detox from sugar or narcotics many times in 1 week.

Your body would reset metabolic food chains and begin the healing of your body. Food is medicine.

Dr. Richard Johnson recommends a 2-week detox and I agree with that. This will repair the damage done by a high fructose diet. This will repair the gut, because, after all, fructose, corn syrup for example, punches holes in your intestine, allowing undigested food to get into the bloodstream, causing immune reactions, which make you sick. The detox will quickly repair the fructose enzymes in your liver, which lead to insulin resistance, leptin resistance and fatty liver.

In the long run you would do fine by simply reducing your fructose intake by 30 to 50%, but in the short term, we want to radically change your metabolism as well as educate you as to what the fructose content is in many different foods. Be sure to use the tables of fructose content of foods and restaurants in this book; they are also illustrated in Dr. Richard Johnson's "A Sugar Fix."

Food Stamp Diet

THE PEOPLE USING FOOD STAMPS are, on the average, more overweight than the rest of us. The country is running about 70% overweight. Our leadership doesn't even bring it up and allows more people to develop a high rate of chronic disease and early death. I do a lot of charitable work in my community, including being a sponsor of a large choir and I am very familiar with it and trying to help the best I can. I write books, CDs, DVDs, participate on a TV show and give frequent lectures about the problem and I think am making some difference.

A first reaction might be that good food is more expensive and there isn't enough money. Really? The majority of people on food stamps don't look like they're starving; it's just the opposite. I give cooking classes with a pediatrician, Dr. Gary Verulla, once a month and about 90% of his patients are on food stamps. When I visit his waiting room, I would say 90% of the parents and children are seriously overweight.

We're doing something about it by offering cooking classes and the children just love it. Teaching a child to cook good food makes you a great parent. To take them to a fast food restaurant and not teach them to cook is almost child abuse. Many parents and their children are blind to the problem. Health care providers must set an example, teach the parents and children and set a good example. People are shopping for quantity and not quality because I don't think they know the difference. Health education in the schools is poor.

A pediatrician walked with me through Wal-Mart, Meijer, Kroger's and some other food markets and I agree that healthy fast food, when properly selected, purchased in larger quantities and prepared properly is clearly cheaper than the alternative. I wish we would have a federal law telling us what is wholesome food with a green, yellow or red light. Whole Foods labels its food with the aggregate nutrient density index (ANDI Score), invented by pediatrician Dr. Joel Fuhrman. I think that's great. But I think a green, yellow and red light would be simpler.

We are slowly killing ourselves. It is better not try to micromanage other people's diets, said the director of an interfaith organization. Dead wrong! It's a public health problem, as Dr. Lustig and many others are recognizing.

The WIC program, a nutrition program for very young children, does have some restrictions on what type of food they can buy with it. It needs to be put across the rest of the food stamp programs. President Obama, please step up to bat. Trying to restrict food choices that are killing us probably will start a food fight. The trouble is some counties in Texas have 40% of the people on food stamps. There is a lot of politics involved. But we are paying the taxes and should have some say.

We need to pass some public health laws, with restrictions on trans fats, fat and sugar content.

Dump the Dairy

OF THE WORLD'S 5,400 MAMMALS, each one produces specially designed milk for its infants. Each type of milk is different when it comes to the amount of protein, carbohydrates and fat.

Why would we want to drink the milk of a cow, which contains 57 hormones, pesticides and herbicides? No other mammal drinks the milk of another mammal, except for humans.

The enzymes we need to digest the lactose in milk decrease significantly by age 4 and 70% of people are born without the ability to digest milk properly. Asians lack the enzyme to break down lactose in milk, 75% of African-Americans are also missing the enzyme. Only 50% of white people have that enzyme.

Infants need mother's milk for good health and metabolism and great brain growth. It supplies the good omega-3 fats.

Cow's milk, however, is unnecessary in the human diet. The U.S. Department of Agriculture's "My Plate" recommends 3 glasses of low-fat milk a day. That's just plain wrong and not good for children's health. The rate of type 1 diabetes is higher in children who drink cow's milk, and there are many allergies associated with lactose, including infections. Many people's gastrointestinal tracts do not tolerate casein, the protein in milk.

A lot of disease occurs because of that, which can be completely avoided.

Without lactase, lactose remains undigested, fermenting in your intestine and causing an array of gastrointestinal symptoms that we refer to as lactose intolerance. Even if your body can break down lactose, it's still bad news, because it is converted to galactose and glucose which elevates blood sugar, causes inflammation and insulin resistance.

Casein, the protein in milk, can prove toxic and eventually lead to neurodegenerative diseases, including attention deficit disorder.

You don't need calcium from milk to keep your bones strong and ward off osteoporosis. Plants have plenty of calcium and are a better source for it. Incidentally, high animal meat protein diets will make the blood acidic, leaching calcium out of the bones in attempt to make the blood more alkaline.

Green leafy vegetables, vitamin D supplements, exercise and increased protein from vegetables are more effective ways for your body to get the calcium it needs.

There are some other reasons for not drinking milk. Milk is generally pasteurized, a heating process to kill bacteria which also kills most of the enzymes that may have made milk slightly worth drinking. It renders milk relatively useless, nutritionally speaking. Cows are generally given growth hormones, which stimulates your liver to produce insulin growth factor, which increases the rate of breast, colon and prostate cancer. These growth hormones are suspected of contributing to early puberty in children. The increase rate of cancer in both children and adults who drink a lot of milk is especially concerning.

Dr. Veerula and Dr. Fuhrman have noticed a tremendous reduction in illness, including infections, allergies, type I diabetes and cancer in their patients who don't drink milk. They say that milk is "liquid meat" and do not recommend it.

History of the Mediterranean diet

WHAT IS IT? HOW GOOD is it?

Many cardiologists recommended it and many nutritionists recommend it.

But has it been tested with double blind clinical studies? Or just epidemiological studies?

Generally the major recommendations include getting most of the energy from vegetables, fruits, legumes and whole grains, seafood, yogurt, nuts, eggs and cheese, red meat rarely and milk never, round out the diet. Olive oil is recommended in abundance.

In the United States, many medical providers recommended this popular diet, as do many cookbooks.

Recent studies have revealed that it's better than a low-fat diet, which has been recommended by cardiologists for 50 years, including the U.S. government. Generally, the Mediterranean diet is a 30 to 40% fat diet. But is it actually nutritionally good for you?

There is a difference between the Mediterranean diet of yesteryear and more recent times. The use of olive oil we've been led to believe goes back a few thousand years. The actual truth is that it only goes back about 200 years, if that.

The real Mediterranean way of eating with real bread, that weighs up to 5 pounds a loaf, has existed in Greece, Italy and Spain for many years, but it is not the Mediterranean diet recommended by nutritionists, doctors, the scientific community and government agencies at this time. The present-day Mediterranean diet is a new invention.

It was invented in the mid-1980s. 2 smart scientists, one from Italy and one from Greece, promoted it and eventually got the job done with the help of many other people.

That may be news to you as it was to me and they made a big difference.

They considered that the traditional Mediterranean way of eating might protect against obesity and heart disease. Clearly, as far as they were concerned, the low-fat way of eating was not working.

Antonio Trichopoulis, a professor at the University of Athens medical school, is known as the "godmother" of the Mediterranean diet, having done more than anyone else to make the diet popular.

As a young medical doctor at the University of Athens medical school, she was advising her patients with high cholesterol to eat various vegetable oils, since that is what the World Health Organization, WHO, following the footsteps of the American Heart Association, had been recommending as a way to stay clear of saturated fats in the fight against heart disease.

Trichopoulis felt compelled to act when she saw olive trees being cut down and the traditional way of life disappearing.

She became aware of the place of olive oil is the diet when patients were telling her they were told to replace them with other vegetable oils, the ones containing omega-6 oils instead of omega-3 oils. Many families had cultivated small plots of olive oil. I once took a train ride over 4 hours to the Spain countryside, enjoying the sight of so many orchards of olive trees, mile after mile.

Yet, due to the global influence of the U.S.-led nutrition policy, which found polyunsaturated oils such as corn, safflower, and soybean oil, the consumption of olive oil in Spain and Greece was dropping.

The bread they were eating no longer weighed 5 pounds, they were eating more sugary bread, and they were continuing to cut down olive trees, which really upset Trichopolous.

She wondered, could olive oil be part of a number of things that protect against vascular disease?

In the 1950s, when Greece was consuming the real Mediterranean way of eating, their life expectancy was number 2 in the world. Denmark was number one.

She started looking at the research of Dr. Ancel Keys from Minnesota. Dr. Keys actually studied 22 countries with U.S. government support money, but reported only on 7. He wanted to promote his saturated fat theory of the causation of heart disease.

He was drawn to the island of Crete and Greece largely because of their residents' longevity. The Cretes appeared to be champions of health.

Keys left a chilling cold state to visit a warm climate Italy and Greece. Eventually he moved south to Sicily on the Mediterranean and died there at age 100. His nutritional research was to become the foundation of the Mediterranean diet.

Crete was cited again and again in research supporting the key secret of a long life. Many medical conferences financed by the olive oil industry happily endorse the Mediterranean diet, based on the experience of researchers who traveled to this area.

If you didn't write a good article for the newspapers for medical journals, you were not invited back.

The 7 country study was published in 1970, although Keys did not identify a Mediterranean diet at that time.

Ultimately the promotion of the Mediterranean diet can about from other scientists and researchers – Trichopoulus especially.

She started studying the diet further in the mid-1980s and began organizing scientific conferences on the Mediterranean diet in Greece.

In Athens the conference gave rise to a lot of scientific papers (diet and nutritional) from professionals and scientists.

In Italy at the same time, Anna Ferro-Luzzi was doing the same thing.

She has been instrumental in the nutrition field in Italy since the 1960s.

She conducted studies on the effect of olive oil in the Mediterranean diet.

She said the diet was very noticeable and hoped to demonstrate that the Mediterranean diet prevented heart disease.

In France and Spain they eat twice as many potatoes than Greece. The French ate more butter. Meat and dairy are more common in the northern countries.

In 1989 Ferro published a landmark paper on the nutrient patterns on most countries bordering the Mediterranean Sea. She concluded it was an impossible enterprise.

She wrote that the Mediterranean diet should not be used in scientific literature until the various nutrients were better defined.

Low-fat diet

SO EVENTUALLY THE LOW-FAT DIET of Ancel Keys ran into the low-fat diet of the American Heart Association, McGovern committee, USDA and the American Heart, Lung, and Blood Institute.

How could an olive oil drenched diet triumph in a world dominated by low-fat diet guidelines?

Vegetable dishes in the Mediterranean were flowing in olive oil.

All that oil conflicted with the Western diet guidelines of 20 to 30% fat.

Mark Hegstead a Harvard professor who steered the McGovern committee said, "You can't recommend a high-fat diet."

Trichoupoli spearheaded the drive for the Mediterranean diet: 40% calories and fat – which is actually no more than the fat in the typical Western diet. She ran scientific studies trying to prove the point.

Ferro-Luzzi in Italy said that Italians were eating a 22-27% fat diet. She put a magnifying glass to the Greek diet and said there was very little scientific data proving their point.

The 2 sides hotly debated the issue and some other scientists remarked they literally had to sit between them at scientific meetings or there might have been a fight.

Trichopoli prevailed because she got the Americans involved.

2 people helped her. Greg Drescher from Cambridge, Mass., was the most vigorous promoter of the Mediterranean diet worldwide. In addition, Walter C. Willett, a professor of epidemiology at the Harvard School of Public Health, played a role in this ongoing debate. Keys would become famous because of his recommended low-fat diet and Walter Willett because of this work on the Mediterranean diet. Dr. Walter Willett had made 2 famous previous recommendations that were both wrong; one was the need for estrogen supplements for women after menopause and the other was a recommendation of vitamin E. Both turned out to be scientifically incorrect.

Drescher and Willett traveled to Athens in the late 1980s to meet Trichopoli. Eventually Drescher and Willett joined forces and they realize that a high-fat diet wrapped in the beauty of the Mediterranean had strong appeal.

Willett and his team eventually designed the Mediterranean diet pyramid. He used only the data from Crete and southern Italy. The data from France, Portugal, Spain and northern Italy wasn't used because it didn't fit his ideas. That is not very scientific and was a mistake, in my opinion.

They thought the people of Crete and southern Italy ate in a similar manner and were generally free of heart disease. They agreed to a 40% fat diet but favored vegetable oils not olive oil, which I think was a major mistake.

In 1993 they had a large conference with 150 experts, carefully selected and controlled from Europe and the United States, to discuss the Mediterranean diet. Even Ancel Keys was there.

The USDA had invented its own pyramid with bread, cereal, rice and pasta at the bottom: a low fat and high carbohydrate diet. Yes, a high sugar diet, wrong again. Olive oil was given a small play in the U.S. diet and a much bigger role in the eventual Mediterranean diet pyramid when published.

The Mediterranean pyramid at the bottom with the largest representation recommended breads grains, including pasta, rice, couscous, polenta and so on. The top of the pyramid with the smallest recommendations was lean red meat, cheese, yogurt and dairy in the middle.

No scientific clinical trials and evaluation had been done of the Mediterranean diet. Ferro-Luzzi from Italy also found it difficult to run studies of significance in her clinical trials in Italy.

The Journal article that Willett's team wrote about the pyramid had poor peer review.

The findings of the conference were published in the American Journal of Clinical Nutrition and guess what? They were paid for by the olive oil industry.

They then moved from science to policy. They publicized the Mediterranean pyramid all over the world and tried to connect it to good health. It frankly went viral. The New York Times wrote 650 articles about it. Considering its connection to Harvard University and many carefully selected scientists, despite their being no clinical trials, it was adopted by many clinicians and people. That the Mediterranean diet was backed by Harvard professors had a great influence.

The method was designed by many research food writers and health authorities attending conferences that were held in paradise, the Mediterranean area. They would travel free of charge to some sun-kissed country and around the gorgeous Mediterranean. If you didn't write a favorable article about the Mediterranean diet, than you were not invited back. You rubbed elbows with chefs, journalists and public officials. Scientific proof was irrelevant.

In retrospect the whole affair with the Mediterranean diet has the most influence nutritionally and everyone was involved, including nutritionists, scientists, providers, the American Heart Association and so on.

The meetings were funded 100% by the government, "Old Ways," the olive oil industry etc. In addition, the Greek government and Spain governments were involved. There were lavish perks aimed at buying good opinions.

Looking back a gentleman named Nestlé, the author of a book called "Food Politics" recognized that the conferences were nothing more than a racket.

The Americans welcomed olive oil because it allowed some fat. The diet swept into cookies, muffins and the American kitchen.

Vegetables, fruit and a new twist: olive oil.

Yet, there remains the question, is it compatible with good health?

What does olive oil have to do with it? Kissed by the sun, the Harvard-endorsed Mediterranean diet had hit the big time.

Americans were now eating more vegetables, fruits, olive oil, more fish, and more nuts. Yet, the general population is still becoming more obese and developing more of its secondary chronic diseases of heart disease, cancer, strokes, autoimmune disease etc. Americans were cooking more with olive oil, getting away from polyunsaturated oils of sunflower, soybean, corn oil and so on. Olive oil consumption tripled.

We began to understand that sunflower oil, soybean oil, and corn oil oxidize easily and can cause free radical damage to our molecules, which are the etiology of a lot of our chronic diseases. Olive oil is more stable, and has only one double bond. I don't think people realize that the Mediterranean diet is a 30 to 40%

fat diet and it is difficult to lose weight when you are using a lot of oil.

Was switching from a low-fat diet to a high-fat diet healthy?

Let's look back at the science. What about the beautiful men in Crete? Is that the olive oil? Is it the exercise, the walking, the socialization and how much animal products they are actually consuming? The data from the studies were from a very small group of people and may not have scientific basis.

The ancient Greeks use olive oil to anoint the body; they didn't use it for food until about 150 years ago. Hippocrates recommended it for G.I. upset as a medicine but not as a staple in the diet.

Fera-Luzzi studied olive oil in Italy and in Greece, including a study of cholesterol levels, which we now know are generally irrelevant to vascular health. She found the LDL level went down 19% over a 6-week period under a controlled study. She wondered if the nutrients in the skin of olives were responsible for this change.

A quick study was done by Dr. Antonio Trichipoli of 20,000 people with volunteers. She published that in the New England Journal of Medicine in 2003 and said overall mortality was reduced on the Mediterranean diet. The study was reviewed by other scientists who noted that olive oil intake was not recorded in the article. Therefore scientists did not know what she got her conclusion from.

Tricopoli couldn't sell the FDA on the science of it and it would not approve labeling that olive oil was healthy.

A Spanish research team in 2011 said there was not much scientific evidence for the Mediterranean diet.

In ancient history Houma called olive oil liquid gold. He meant it was best in a gold container, which was discovered by Dr. Nina

Teicholtz, who wrote "The Big Fat Surprise" when she reviewed the famous publication "The Iliad." Ancient people used olive oil as a cosmetic and not as a food.

Ancel Keys said we have been using it for 4,000 years but 150 years or so is more accurate. Olive oil was used a lot for soap in the 19th century.

So what is it that results in better health for the people on the island of Crete? They walk a lot; I was there playing a tennis tournament and saw this firsthand, they eat a lot of more vegetables and fruit, they don't eat dessert unless it's a fruit. Very little pie or cake. I visited a Greek restaurant recently, I realize this is not Greece, and to me the food was inedible, full of fat and sugar and the customers unfortunately looked accordingly, including a child who was sitting at the next table, which concerned me a great deal. A teenager with a huge potbelly. Remember this is a no-judgment zone. I'm extremely concerned about the child's future as a physician and caring person.

The point is that using 2 tablespoons of olive oil, full of omega-3, the good essential fatty acid, may have some value, although the scientific proof is sparse. Remember all vegetable oils are hundred percent fat and are very fattening if you use them a lot.

When Walter Willett unveiled the Mediterranean pyramid, no clinical trial had been done.

Trichopoli combined data from Greek and European studies of 75,000 males and females, and the Mediterranean diet was not reliably associated with a reduction in coronary risk.

Then she developed the Mediterranean diet index, which includes eight factors with one point for each recommendation.
- a-vegetarian/potatoes
- b-legumes-nuts c-fruits d-none processed cereals

- one point each with a maximum of 4
- Increase ratio of olive oil/animal fats-one point
- low use of dairy products-one point
- low rate of dairy consumption-one point
- low rate of meat and poultry consumption
- low rate of alcohol use-one point, total of 3 points possible

The index didn't work very well. Mother Greece was favored over science. They were thinking with their heart and the evidence from science was not that good.

There was a large study done in France called the Lyon study, named after the city. It was quite small but much quoted. It didn't even use olive oil, but used margarine instead.

The problems are described in a paper by the American Heart Association, which was in an awkward position, trying to recover from its own low-fat diet recommendations. Patients were actually doing better with high-fat diets.

A test of the real Mediterranean diet was done in 2008 in Israel. It was well-designed and rigorous by a good group of scientists. The group included Eir Stampfer of the Harvard School of Public Health.

They studied 322 moderately obese people. They placed them on the low carbohydrate, low-fat diet, and the Mediterranean diet for 2 years. They made them use the same cafeteria.

The ones who ate the Mediterranean diet had increase HDL, lower triglycerides, lower LDL, lower CRP and a lower insulin level.

The low carbohydrate group with increased fat consumption did the best and looked the healthiest. They had reduced triglycerides and increased HDL. They lost the most weight.

In 2013 a large study came from Spain and was thought to solve the problem of evaluating the Mediterranean diet. It was called the Predimed Study. They divided them into 3 groups and studied them for 5 years.

The study demonstrated that the Mediterranean diet is better than the low-fat diet, but not as good as the low carbohydrate diet. Olive oil consumption may not have had much to do with it.

Maybe any diet is better than the AHA-USDA diet.

Only 33 men were studied in Crete and 34 on Corfu. So the Mediterranean diet the study made by Keys only covered very small groups. Don't you wonder how many people may have been injured, became sick or died from the low fat recommendation?

Sugar has been swept under the rug. Dr. Keys is dead but the American Heart Association, the US Lung and Heart Institute, the USDA, and many scientists who recommended the low-fat diet are still around. I think they should speak up but I just don't think it's going to happen. Such a small sample size was in no way representative of the 8.7 million Greeks, and 440,000 Cretes.

The scientific information was passed along by the community without good clinical studies then Walter Willett from Harvard built his Mediterranean pyramid.

They left milk off the pyramid, although the Greeks were drinking a good glass a day. They were also historically eating a lot more meat than was represented in the Keys and Willett data.

Another historical inaccuracy of the Mediterranean diet is the absence of red meat. The Grecians actually preferred red meat: goat, beef and mutton and some chicken. On the island of Corfu, they ate beef and veal.

Dr. Willet wrote that low consumption of red meat was a hallmark of the Mediterranean diet. That actually was not true, most the time they were starving and just couldn't afford it. Picking chicken as the main meat has no basis in the history of the Mediterranean diet. Willett picked chicken because he felt red meat was unhealthy.

It appears in following the Mediterranean diet we are relying on data collected by Keys in postwar Greece from a handful of men, partially during Lent, the religious holiday, and then distorted by Dr. Willet, who as biased against fat consumption to begin with.

Perhaps the paradox can be explained by the evil twins-sugar and fructose. Greeks don't eat sugary desserts very much. There is nearly a complete absence of sugary foods. It's not the fat problem but the toxic sugar. Cake is seldom served and pie almost never.

Should we all be Mediterranean? Olive oil, which is 100% fat, will certainly lead to weight gain. 2 tablespoons certainly can be tolerated. Certainly the Mediterranean diet has given some relief to the low-fat diets, and it's a good deal better than polyunsaturated oils of soybeans, corn, safflower and especially oxidized vegetable oils. The diet is helping us to get over the fear of animal fats but that can be a problem, too. After all we need to be able to tell the difference between organic and nonorganic meat production, the latter being full of inflammatory essential fatty acids, pesticides herbicides and genetically altered corn.

Early Diagnosis

THERE IS A LOT OF controversy here. Opinion frankly carries the day. Decades old double-blind studies of nutrition and eating habits are hard to find. Forty-4 years of experience in the field should have some value.

Common sense is the king here.

The HRA, health risk assessment, should be number one. That should begin in childhood. Exactly what age? That would depend on family history or if the child has unusual early onset of obesity. If grandparents, siblings or mother or father have significant metabolic illnesses or death at a young age, then biometric, blood tests should be run as early as age 2. The rate of obesity is actually accelerating in the 2- to 6-year age range. The sooner you correct the problem, the easier it will be. Eating habits honestly become more difficult to correct the longer they have been there.

Blood work will be abnormal before obesity sets in, but not always. Children should have their weight and height checked at least once a year and more so with a strong family history. If both parents are overweight, then the child has a 70% chance of being overweight. If one parent has a weight problem, than it ought to run around 30 to 40%. Generally, many providers don't check the biometrics, the blood work of teenagers unless there is a strong family history of chronic disease. Personally, I think that is a mistake. Even if they have a normal BMI, teens should fill out a health risk assessment form and have their biometrics checked. After all we're looking to reduce the rate of this plague tremendously. In the long run it will save tremendous amount of illness and health care dollars.

You need to check the metabolism of the liver after a basic HRA assessment, including:

- NMR-lipid profile: It determines the particle size and number of LDL, HDL and triglycerides. Large amounts of small dense LDL is a sign of trouble. Even normal cholesterol won't tell the story. You need a low density LDL test. You should have fewer than 1,000 LDL particles and less than 500 small LDL particles.
- Liver enzyme test-AST, ALT, GGT-to assess fatty liver
- 2-hour glucose tolerance test
- Serum insulin and blood sugar (1-2 hours of fasting)
- Lipid profile
- Cholesterol: <150
- LDL: <70
- HDL: > 60-female
- HDL: > 50-male
- Triglycerides: <100
- Triglyceride/HDL ratio
- Total cholesterol/HDL ratio
- Hemoglobin A1c
- Gluten panel sensitivity test

An insulin response test is very important to catch early metabolic syndrome or type 2 diabetes,

This test measures your insulin and blood sugar at the same time. This will help providers catch the majority of metabolic diseases very early when it is much easier to correct them.

The test measures glucose and insulin levels after a 75 gram gross load. Your blood sugar can be normal but you insulin could be sky high. I saw this many times in my practice.

That is why diabesity, diabetes and obesity, is not diagnosed early in 90% of people who have it. You can see why this is so critical. Look at the tremendous amount of disease we misdiagnose.

If you have abnormal lab tests, they should be repeated at least every 3 months while you are taking corrective action. The provider should see you frequently, otherwise get a new provider or insist on more frequent tests.

To assess the severity of complications if you have abnormal metabolic test and it is clear you have a problem, then you need to get additional blood tests. If you would like to use the Internet, take advantage of Dr. Mark Hyman's excellent website. I also recommend his book "The Blood Sugar Solution." You can download it at www.bloodsugarsolution.drhyman.com.

If we are going to stop this epidemic, we need to start very early.

Not everyone would agree. If 20 to 40% of people with normal weight have abnormal biometric liver testing, then according to Dr. Mark Hyman, we need to do regular biometric testing. This is the future. It is a lot easier to take corrective action at a young age. If we miss disease for up to a decade, then that person is missing out on years of their life.

We spend $2.7 trillion on health care yearly; we could reduce this by $1 trillion if we take more early action. Right now we have "sick care."

Obese teenagers should be treated aggressively while we still have a chance at changing their habits.

Everyone should exercise at least 30 minutes per day.

Although we don't hear a lot of great things about the English health care system, they practice preventative healthcare big time. Almost all patients have their biometrics tested on a yearly basis because they have found it to be highly preventative. The doctor's offices are full of signs promoting wellness such as phone numbers to call for additional help. The family doctor gets paid more for keeping you well. You will notice when you travel in Europe that obesity is not much of a problem. When Europeans come here, they are shocked by the size of our population. We badly need to create a culture of wellness, and number one on that paradigm is that the patient must participate in his or her healthcare. In addition, providers need to participate by teaching every patient when the opportunity arises. For example, I have CDs, DVDs and TV shows and take the time to coach most patients in spite of a very busy schedule. I've been doing this for more than 30 years. I also write books and they're all on Amazon. The majorities are about wellness from every angle.

In summary I highly recommend really persistent, repeated health risk assessment and biometric testing as the best way to turn the United States healthcare crisis around.

Prevention through Fitness

EXERCISE HAS BEEN PROVEN TO be a huge component of health since ancient times. Look at the Greek and Roman Coliseums. Athletes were worshiped.

We've been promoting it to the public for 2 centuries.

Hippocrates, a physician in the 4th century BC, placed a lot of emphasis on prevention of illness. He recognized that natural living was the road to good health and involved regular exercise.

It was called "hygiene," a Greek word for health, embracing all the activities relative to health over which a person has control.

So practicing good wellness habits is actually demonstrating your "hygiene" in Greek terms.

Hygiene has been narrowed to mean cleanliness, but for the most of our history it meant all the things you could do to insure vitality and health.

At the beginning of the Industrial Revolution, we became more sedentary and started doing less physical labor.

Time and time again, a poor city dweller was contrasted with a farmer. And the health statistics proved that. The stockbroker versus the farmer.

Health promoters since the 1800s recommended the system of exercise and diet.

In the 1830s a populist health reform movement was started by Sylvester Graham, a minister. It was called "Grahamism." He demonized alcohol and meat from animals. He is responsible for the Graham cracker and he also recommended a vegetarian diet.

Strenuous physical exercise was strongly recommended, running over walking.

Another movement in the later part of the 1800s was called "muscular Christianity."

It had a profound cultural impact, elevating building strength and endurance to an act of faith. It was considered a spiritual duty to stay healthy. By the end of the 1860s, he who neglected the body was considered to be committing a sin.

The German system of exercise called Turnin gymnastics was brought to the United States in the 1820s. This incorporated strength, bending and weightlifting including dumbbells, but was not popular.

Then the new gymnastics was brought forth called the Lewis system, a formal physical exercise promoted throughout the country. The Lewis system was rapidly adapted across the country in schools and colleges.

In the 1860s the country turned to the strength-building program of George Winship. After signing up for medical school at Harvard, he invented a system of weight machines and gave lectures all over the country focusing on strength and health; he started a weight lifting mania.

Dudley Allen Sargent developed the Sargent system of weight training, using full weight machines at Harvard. It was adapted by 250 colleges, 300 public school systems and 500 YMCAs. People got tired of machines and we started participating more in team sports. You can imagine, though, that left a lot of children behind and many are still left out today. Most of the country is watching things, sitting on a couch eating bad food and not participating.

In the 1900s we concentrated on infectious diseases because they caused most of our illnesses and deaths.

In World War I and in recent wars, about 50% of the recruits did not pass a physical. Actually about 75% of today's children are not physically fit.

In 1963 President John F. Kennedy took a step in the right direction by promoting the Council on Physical Fitness, which is still operating in most of the schools in the country.

Jack LaLanne, "the Godfather of fitness," promoted physical fitness for more than 70 years. He died at age 96 having lived a full life without illness.

In addition to strength training, yoga, tai chi, Zumba dancing, walking, running and swimming are all great forms of exercise than can improve physical and mental fitness.

Planet Fitness where I work out daily should be congratulated. They dropped the price to $9.99 per month. So now almost anybody can afford to work out. Personally, I think this should be part of every insurance plan. The above facility where I work out has 9,000 members; I think 5 million in the country. It makes me smile every day.

Infectious diseases were the biggest cause of death in the 1800s and first half of the 1900s. But now we look at the complications of what we are eating, lack of exercise, stress and more; we have a 75% adult obesity rate, and a 30% children's obesity rate.

The majority of diseases such as type 2 diabetes, hypertension, half of the various types of cancer, autoimmune disease and stress can be avoided with proper eating, exercise, stress reduction and strength training. We could reduce all chronic diseases by 80% and probably save $1 trillion in healthcare costs. I spoke to a 4th year medical student yesterday and she said, she had one hour of nutrition education in her 4 years of medical school. She'll be a doctor and study pediatrics by July! How do you spell "pathetic", "sad"?

What do I recommend?

First I think you need a basic understanding of your risk factors from your healthcare provider.

Exercise should be done by children, causing it to become a habit. It can't just be e-mail, texting, TV and watching team sports. I'm now 77 years old and exercise 90 minutes every day, and I did so even as a child living in New York City in Central Park. I worked 44 years as a neurosurgeon day and night and still managed to find the time to exercise. Either get up early or go to bed late or figure something out that matches your situation, because it is critical to your health. Exercise improves your metabolism and helps you avoid those chronic diseases. Exercise will generally not cause that much weight loss, eating the right food is a better way to keep your weight under control. My father lived to be 89 years old, my mother 97; they did it with a fatty German deli diet but they worked hard and walked daily a lot and didn't smoke, and the food was organic.

Since ancient times, yoga, tai chi and chi gong have combined stretching, breathing techniques, meditation and visualization to promote good physical and mental health.

They guide individuals through a set of motions to improve strength, balance and self-confidence. Western countries usually include flexibility exercises as part of the strengthening and aerobic workout routines. I highly recommend that.

Flexibility is the extent to which certain tissues in the body can change safely and comfortably. Flexibility decreases with age.

Inactivity fosters "cross-links" or binding of the proteins that can close off muscles, tendons and ligaments. These cross-links are reversible.

A stretch of 15 seconds is adequate.

The health benefits of exercise for people at risk of developing or having diabetes include:

- Improves glycemic control
- Increases metabolism and promotes weight loss
- Reduces risk of metabolic syndrome
- Improves insulin sensitivity
- Improves blood pressure
- Inhibits diseases such as heart disease, strokes, cancer and autoimmune disease
- Reduces stress and depression
- Increases muscular strength and size
- Increase neuroplasticity (grow your brain)

Dr. Franklin House feels intermittent training is the key to increasing physical activity among sedentary Americans. It is non-continuous activity that incorporates active rest for a fraction of a minute of moderate activity. I do that all the time. Walk moderately fast followed by walking slow on the treadmill, for example, for at least 5 to 10 repetitions. This will improve your reserve of your heart. You make your body work a little, then you let it rest a little, then you make it work again and so on. You do this by exercising 5 heartbeats above your target heart rate and then 5 beats below your target heart rate. You don't stop the activity completely; you slow down enough to rest. For example, you jog, and then you walk. The added benefits of intermittent training include greater weight loss and body fat loss.

Energy for activity comes in 2 basic metabolic sources, oxygen metabolism and anaerobic muscle metabolism. Aerobic fitness is a large burst of energy in a short period of time; sprinting or heavy lifting would qualify. You may go into anaerobic metabolism within about 3 minutes of exercise. The intensity of the activity exceeds the ability of the heart and lungs to get oxygen to the muscles being worked. But what is the gold standard of health, fitness and well-being? It's your VO2 max that counts. Anaerobic activity uses glycogen, a form of sugar stored within muscle cells.

Find your target heart rate and use it to train. Subtract your age in years from 220, then take that number multiplied by .65 and that is your target heart rate. Your training zone will be 5 beats slower and 5 beats higher than your target heart rate.

Frankly, walking a mile a day 5 days a week, fast slow, fast slow, depending on ability, plus lifting reasonable weights for 10 to 15 minutes 3 times a week, preceded by 5 minutes of stretching is good enough for most people. If you are eating good food, you will live to be 100.

It's your HRA, health risk assessment, your biometrics, the blood tests, exercise history, and what type of food you eating that will determine your health most of the time. Certainly genes can play a role but generally they will not express themselves unless you have bad eating habits and challenge your evolutionary genetic history. Genes play at best a 10 to 15% role in overall health.

Remember your HRA and biometric tests and your exercise routine above all. Also, get that 2-hour glucose tolerance test and serum insulin and blood sugar at an early age and periodically repeat it.

Taking Back Our Health

WE'RE HAVING A NATIONAL AND international epidemic of obesity, type 2 diabetes, heart disease, vascular disease, strokes and cancer. The China Study by Dr. Colin Campbell certainly pointed us in that direction. The United States has the second-highest rate of obesity in the world, only second to Mexico. It's about fat, salt and sugar, with sugar being the main culprit.

Each year, Americans suffer 1.5 million heart attacks, including 850,000 deaths from heart attacks, 35 million people have type 2 diabetes, and 125 million people have metabolic syndrome, in addition to some of the highest rates of cancer in the world and essentially leading the world in chronic disease. 75 percent of us are overweight, 35 to 40% are obese, one third of our children are overweight -- from those figures, and you can predict the future.

This is a no judgment zone; I'm just trying to help solve the problem that is killing us.

High Fructose Foods

HIGH FRUCTOSE FOODS INCLUDE CANDY, cookies, cakes, pies, and other baked goods, fruit, fruit juice and other beverages that contain fruit, honey, sports drinks, soda and other soft drinks. You must become very conscious as to what the fructose content of food is and start reading labels. Especially avoid high fructose corn syrup, but then again all fructose is dangerous.

There are many variations of the terms sucrose or table sugar: beet sugar, brown sugar, cane sugar, corn sweetener, corn syrup, maple syrup, glasses, raw sugar, sucrose, table sugar, etc.

Eliminating food from your diet for 2 weeks means you may be missing some important nutrients. For this reason, I recommend taking some supplements for a few weeks: a multivitamin with minerals, plus 50 mg of vitamin C.

Consider avoiding restaurants and take-out food during the fructose free phase, because it's hard to be certain if the food you're ordering contains sugar or high fructose corn syrup. You should drink 5 cups of water per day. If you need to drink alcohol, consume only one glass of wine a day or less.

Trans fatty acids

THEY ARE TRANSFORMED BY ADDING one hydrogen atom into vegetable oils. They cannot be properly metabolized by the liver and are a great threat to your health. They increase your low density LDL, the one that digs into your lining of your blood vessels to cause atherosclerosis, heart disease and strokes. A doughnut, for example, may be 35 to 40% trans fatty acids, a killer. One-reason restaurants and markets like these products is that they don't rot.

Feedlot animal meat including beef, pork, lamb, chicken, turkey and fish (when raised on a farm) are a source of the Omega-6, AA, arachidonic acids, versus ocean fish which is full of the anti-inflammatory Omega-3; organic-raised animal meats have more Omega-3.

Fat is metabolically very active and produces some nasty chemicals. Abdominal fat is more dangerous than fat on your hips, since abdominal fat is in your liver, pancreas and bowel and not just under your skin. It's very metabolically active. About 25% of the people in this nation have infiltration of the liver by fat. It causes scarring of the liver and interferes with its function. The latter results in insulin resistance, diabetes and more; most people do not know that they have a fatty liver, they may even be of normal weight.

The shape of the body and where the fat is located make a difference. If you are apple-shaped, you are more likely to have fatty liver disease. Non-alcoholic fatty liver disease will be the most common cause of liver transplants in the future and not cirrhosis from alcoholism.

How can you tell if you're overweight? This is important to know because 80% of the people who are overweight have metabolic syndrome and will develop significant chronic diseases like heart disease, vascular disease, strokes, cancer, autoimmune disease and dementia. So prevention is critical.

There are a number of ways to tell if you're overweight besides the visual estimate:

- Neck measurement: This is not well known but is the most accurate, check tables on the Internet.
- BMI-body mass index: Check tables and books and Internet
- Dexa scan
- MRI or ultrasound
- Pelvic-umbilicus ratio measurement

By age 2, we have 90% of our fat cells. How much we will weigh at birth is a lot of genetics and parents' habits. Then during intrauterine development, the weight of the child will be determined a great deal by the pre- and pregnancy habits of the mother. Is she smoking, is she taking drugs, what is she eating? My daughter had a baby recently and I reminded her to eat a lot of vegetables during her pregnancy. My 2-year-old grandson looks just great.

Foods with a lot of trans fatty acids include biscuits, cookies, cream, crackers, donuts, fried foods, margarine and potato chips.

Obesity in our children is due in great part to the industrialization of food, fast food restaurants, plus ever-increasing combinations of fat, salt and sugar being served to us. The government is part of the conspiracy because they support the price of fat, salt and sugar to make food cheaper so we buy more of it. It's a combination of the industry and the government. Chicken McNuggets have 39 ingredients, many of them fat, salt and sugar; McDonalds then adds a spray so that they taste like chicken.

We are born with a taste for salt, sweet, bitterness and sour. We have no fat taste buds. You have to teach your child to eat fat. We have receptors for sugar throughout our mouth, tongue, and hard palate and all the way down the esophagus.

Is the U.S. Department of Agriculture interested in your health? If you visit the USDA in Washington D.C., you would find a huge department at the center of town. If you wanted to visit the nutrition office, the one that worries about your health, you would have to take a subway ride under the Potomac River, then take a bus ride, then walk one-third of a mile and take an elevator to the 7th floor in a building at the edge of Alexandria, Virginia. This small office supposedly helps to promote and protect your health. Who do you think has the upper hand here: the food companies or government officials? Or you, the public? Let's not kid each other: we the people are irrelevant. It's the industry lobby with its money and the guys with their hand out who keep themselves in office to get the nice pensions and the best health-care policies in the country. We the people pay the price with a shorter lifespan and many chronic illnesses. We need restrictions on the salt, fat and sugar content of food. The least we could do is tax the fat, salt and sugar and apply the money to health care.

We spend $1 trillion a year on food, and $2.7 trillion on health care, or let's call it "sick care."

Sugar is our methadone; it gets us on a high very quickly and makes us feel great. It affects the serotonin and dopamine circuitry in the brain. Fat is the opiate, a smooth operator whose affect is less obvious but no less powerful.

The molecules make us feel great like amphetamines, narcotics, sex, gambling, alcohol and cigarettes. The brain chemistry is exactly the same. A lot of people say food is more addictive than cocaine. This has been proven on functional MRI scanners. Ice cream lights up the scanner like an A-bomb.

The Cargill Corporation makes 17 sweeteners, 40 types of salt, and 21 oils and fats.

In 1999 about 10 CEOs of the largest food producers and manufacturers met at a hotel to discuss the increasing obesity problem. They fully agreed it was there, and a reporter dug out the information, although this meeting was supposed to be completely secret. The industry decided to do nothing about it and said, in essence, "We don't give a damn. It's only profits that count."

Fat is energy dense and is 9 calories per gram, versus sugar and protein, which are 4 calories a gram.

Cheese is the largest source of saturated fat. Cheese is generally 50 to 80% fat, and we consume 33 pounds of cheese a year, plus 133 pounds of sugar year.

Whole milk is 3% fat, and one glass of whole milk has 225 calories, 7.5 g of saturated fat. No mammals drink the milk of another mammal except humans. Of course, mother's milk is a healthy thing and newborn children should drink it because of the good essential fatty acids. Our brain is 50% Omega-3.

The Kraft food company hired Paula Dean to sell a lot of high-fat sugary foods and help make the nation sick. In particular, she used their cheese in 5,000 recipes, helping the company make millions. Little consideration was given to the health of the public.

I accidentally walked into Paula Dean's restaurant in Savannah, Georgia. I had never heard of her and I didn't look at the sign on the restaurant. The first thing I passed was the fried food line and remember using the words "they should burn this place down" based just on what I was seeing inside the restaurant: many obese people and very nasty food. I did not know where I had been until I told some of the nurses at home this story and they said, "Oh, you must have been at Paula Dean's." Can you just imagine the number of people who became obese and unhealthy because of the food she was selling and advertising? Have you noticed she developed type 2 diabetes a few years ago but didn't tell anyone for years? Isn't it strange that people are not upset about this?

Nonalcoholic fatty liver disease, NAFLD, is a huge problem in this nation, and many people don't know they have it. Unfortunately, a significant number of people of normal weight have fat in their liver. Usually, though, their triglycerides or CRP would be abnormal to give you a hint. Therefore, you should get your biometrics checked even if you are looking good, feeling good and of normal weight.

In summary, to know the distribution of your fats is important no matter what you weigh. Fat, salt and sugar are what's killing us, with sugar the king of all. If you are going to eat some animal products, always know where they came from and eat as low fat as you can. Remember even beef that has all visible fat removed is still 20 to 40% fat, so don't fool yourself. A lot of people think chicken is a healthy food and they're just dead wrong; even without skin, chicken is 20 to 30% fat unless specially prepared.

Sugar and the Brain

OUR ANCESTORS, HUMAN AND ANIMAL, ate fruit with fructose only a few months a year. In addition, the foods they consumed had more fiber than those we consume today.

Fructose is the weakest of all natural sugars. Fructose is low on the glycemic index because it does not stimulate insulin production.

Diabetes has profound effects on the brain because of sugar metabolism. The data regarding diabetes, dementia and Alzheimer's disease is profound. Diabetics also have a powerful risk of cognitive decline and dementia. Avoiding diabetes, especially poor control, is critical. I work a lot with the diabetic doctors, PAs and nurse practitioners who say diabetic patients have only a 50% compliance rate, so you can imagine what the sugars are doing to their body: amputations, heart attacks, strokes, dementia, vascular disease, autoimmune disease and cancer and many other illnesses, including blindness.

A more recent study recently proved a direct link between the rate of cognitive decline and increased levels of HBA 1C.

The combination of sugar and protein in the blood forms a nasty chemical combination called advanced glycation end products (AGE's). Advanced glycation products cause protein in fiber to become misshapen and inflexible. Just look at the type 2 diabetic and a smoker and the older person, those are the visible effects of advanced glycation products. You can predict the aging process in the body by obtaining a blood marker, advanced glycation product and HbA1c.

High fructose corn syrup increases the rate of glycation and formation of AGEs 10 times. You can see the problem. That is a huge statistic.

When protein becomes glycated, it binds to sugar, causes cross protein links, which gum up our vasculature, nerves, brain, eyes, organs, skin, etc. This causes free radicals, oxidation and the rotting and frying of our brain. The best way to reduce AGE formation is proper eating and avoiding the evil twin, fructose.

The bottom line is you want to reduce oxidative stress and the action of free radicals from harming your brain and reduce your aggregated glycation end products.

Avoiding fructose is number one and also glucose because it causes obesity.

Fructose Free for 2 Weeks

WE NEED TO REDUCE THE number of fructose enzymes. We don't eliminate all fructose, because some vegetables and other foods contain a small amount, which is of no consequence to you. Remember, usually you can consume up to 35 grams of fructose a day and be very healthy. The trouble is we are consuming 66 grams a day.

The Problem with Fruit

REMEMBER, FRUIT HAS FRUCTOSE IN it and does not metabolize any differently, to my dismay. Then again, it has a lot of fiber with it and after the first 2-week period, I think it is reasonable to eat 2 or 3 servings a day if your health is improving.

Fructose Metabolism Reviewed

AFTER EATING FRUCTOSE, 100% OF the metabolic burden rests on your liver, as opposed to only 20 percent with glucose.

Every cell in your body, including your brain, utilizes glucose. By contrast, fructose is turned into free fatty acids, VLDL, very low-density LDL, triglycerides that get stored as fat. The fatty acids created during fructose metabolism accumulate as fat droplets in your liver and skeletal muscle tissues, causing insulin resistance and non-alcoholic liver disease, and insulin resistance progresses to metabolic syndrome and type 2 diabetes.

Fructose is the most lipophilic carbohydrate. In addition, fructose converts to activated glycerol, G3 P, which forms free fatty acids, resulting in triglycerides and fat. The more G3 P you have, the more fat you store. Glucose does not do this. Fructose and glucose cause our triglycerides to be high, not fat!

One hundred and twenty calories of fructose results in 40 calories being stored as fat. Consuming fructose is essentially consuming fat! The metabolism of fructose creates a long list of waste products and toxins, including large amounts of uric acid, which drives up blood pressure and causes gout.

Glucose depresses the hunger hormone ghrelin and interferes with your brains communication with leptin, resulting in overeating.

If anyone tries to tell you sugar is just glucose, they're way behind the times. The bottom line is that fructose leads to increased belly fat, insulin resistance and metabolic syndrome, not to mention a long list of chronic diseases. Eating sugar will accelerate the aging process itself.

Artificial Sweeteners

ARTIFICIAL SWEETENERS ARE INCREASINGLY USED to satisfy a sweet tooth. Unfortunately, the only one I recommend is Stevia. It's a natural plant from Mexico and most people think it is quite safe. Stevia leaves are 10 to 15 times sweeter than sugar, although a problem with artificial sweeteners is it will increase your desire for other sweets.

If you are switching from sugar to artificial sweeteners, you are jumping from the frying pan into the fire. That's the opinion of many nutritionists.

Artificial sweeteners actually elevate insulin levels, because they signal to the brain that something sweet is coming even though it is not. The brain secretes hormones that do that. Artificial sweeteners can distort metabolic hormonal messages and trigger hunger, because they provide no calories; the longer this goes on, the more you will eat. Artificial sweeteners are known to cause belly fat and weight gain. Artificial sweeteners also contribute to sugar cravings and sugar addiction, because they are much sweeter than sugar. Also, artificial sweeteners are created by chemical processes that require the use of strong chemicals, which can further harm the body. If you need a sweetener, Stevia the best option, according to many nutritionists. I use nothing and have a 4-pack for a belly. I will be 78 next month!

The International Fat Epidemic

SURVIVAL OF THE FATTEST IS a new paradigm.

There are 1½ billion obese people in the world, and 100 million dying yearly as a result of the complications of heart disease, stroke, type 2 diabetes, cancer, autoimmune diseases and numerous other illnesses. All of this is produced by what's on our spoons and forks and the sugary drinks we consume.

There is an evolutionary fight between our genetic structure and the genes of our food. There has not been enough time over the course of evolution to change our genetic structure to mitigate the threats to our health. It's an equal opportunity employer.

It's occurring throughout the world now. It used to be just the Western societies, but it is spreading like the plague throughout Asia, South Vietnam, South Korea, the Middle East, Europe, the Persian Gulf and especially many of the isolated islands of the Pacific. On one Pacific island, Natur, 95% of the people are obese. It's happening in Africa where they used to eat mainly vegetables and had none of these problems. Some groups are affected more than others based on education, race, poverty and sedentary lifestyle.

The great pandemic of history was the Black Death of the 14th century that killed 45 million people. It was caused by bacteria, yersinia pestis. It killed quickly, in a matter of days.

The Spanish flu of 1918 was also very deadly. It killed 40 million people from a virus within weeks.

The ongoing epidemic we are having from AIDS has been shown to be caused by a virus from mammals in Africa. It's killed about 25 million people so far and 100 million may be infected. The new drugs are helping a great deal.

It is the opinion of Dr. Richard Johnson that the greatest epidemic of all is obesity and its secondary diseases, which have killed so many people over the decades. It's my opinion that obesity will have killed 200 million people a year in another 10 to 15 years and maybe more. It will kill more people than all the other illnesses and epidemics combined. The difference though is the present epidemic can be stopped, prevented and cured.

The *Wall Street Journal* recently carried a great exposé on the obesity and diabetic problem across the world but especially in the Persian Gulf countries. It is caused by lack of exercise, the sugary food and a sedentary lifestyle. Likewise, the *New York Times* ran an expose describing the great increase in obesity surgery on children in the Persian Gulf countries. There wasn't much talk in either article on the food they were eating. Let's face it: If parents didn't feed children sugary foods, the epidemics wouldn't exist. Parents are having the same problem and that complicates matters tremendously. Education is the key.

Dr. James Neal proposed the "Thrifty Gene" hypothesis in 1961. He suggested that the rise in obesity and diabetes observed throughout the world today was due to the genes that we acquired in the past. He points out that the animals and insects had the ability to store fat, and survived because of it. Evolution selected them to be the parents of the future.

The story of hibernation of different living creatures tells the real story. Some frogs can survive 5 years without eating. Whales don't eat while swimming 5,000 kilometers to their place of reproduction in Mexico. The hummingbird stores up to 40% fat in one day from eating sugar. Its liver literally turns white.

Dr. Neil suggests that during periods of famine, those individuals who carried the gene that would favor the greatest accumulation of fat would be more likely to survive. Asians, African-Americans, people in the Persian Gulf and some Americans carry more of these genes and you can see the results if they eat the wrong food. If they eat mainly a plant diet, they are perfectly healthy and thin.

So eating too much and lack of exercise is not the total answer, it's what you are eating.

Some people are just more prone to become overweight if they eat the wrong food. Sugar, especially fructose and saturated fats including polyunsaturated omega-6s, lead to obesity.

Living things, animals, amphibians, insects, etc. even develop insulin resistance when getting ready for hibernation. But when they are done hibernating, the switch is turned off and they get back to their normal weight, within .5%, quickly.

But we humans don't. Some say it's a rheostat and not a switch, we've lost control of the mechanism.

Dr. Richard Johnson feels its loss of the uric acid enzyme, uricase, that's supposed to destroy uric acid and clear it out of the body through the kidneys that is the problem. That was lost thousands of years ago through the process of evolution. Uric acid increases fat deposits, and the only people who didn't have this enzyme lived and were selected throughout evolution for survival. He feels the same thing happened with the ability to make vitamin C. Vitamin C reduces fat deposits, and evolution favored those who didn't have the vitamin C gene. In other words this double knockout of this uricase enzyme and loss of vitamin C increased our propensity to keep the fat switch on. It was a survival mechanism.

Weight is Tightly Controlled in Nature

THE EMPEROR PENGUIN WILL NOT eat for 6 months while the male incubates the egg lying on his feet. He is totally dependent on the fat stored in his abdomen. He has developed insulin resistance. He stored up the fat throughout the summer and is dependent on his fat switch.

The increase in fat is scheduled and regulated by nature. Unfortunately that is not the case in humans. Most wild animals by nature have become periodically obese by evolutionary design. The ones that couldn't do it died out. Animals will switch from fat accumulation, phase 2 of fat burning, on genetic demand. It's highly regulated.

What happened to us? Being fat had a survival advantage in evolution.

Most animals store fat very similar to us. Subcutaneous, liver, bowel, neck, back, buttocks, and abdomen etc., although a recent article indicated that hibernating bears, the grizzly bear specifically, did not store the fat in its organs but under the skin. Interesting. I bet he doesn't have insulin resistance. Seals can weigh up to 3,000 pounds and then fast up to 60 days while swimming to another reproductive site. Humans can go without eating for only about a month.

In hibernation, animals decrease their metabolic rate, reduce their temperature and reduce up to 90% of their usual energy needs. Hibernation is a powerful mechanism of decreasing energy needs. The basic metabolic rate goes way down. You can see how important our basic metabolic rate is when you look at its effect on fat metabolism and energy needs.

Sugar, especially fructose, is accompanied by hypertension, arterial disease, vascular disease, heart attacks, strokes, and cancer and is killing us.

The French physician Etienne Lancereaux, 1829-1891, separated type 1 diabetes, no insulin, from type 2 diabetes, too much insulin. Type 1 patients are lean and type 2 are overweight. But now many advanced type 2 diabetics become lean because they lose the ability to make insulin, their pancreas is dying out and now they have both diseases and soon will be on dialysis, have visual loss, nerve loss, amputations, memory loss etc.? Prevention is the key.

Metabolic syndrome was first described in 1920 and then popularized by Dr. Gerald Raven in the 1980s. Twenty-5 percent of people in the United States have metabolic syndrome. That includes hypertension, and a waistline greater than 40 inches for males and 35 inches for females as well as high triglycerides, greater than 150, high LDL, low HDL and a fasting blood sugar greater than 110. If you have 2 or 3 of these, you have metabolic syndrome. Probably 100 to 250 million people in the United States have it. It's an epidemic here and across the world.

Insulin resistance accompanies the fat storage of hibernation and is in the crosshairs of metabolic syndrome and our obesity story. Animals preparing for food storage turn on the fats, which cause insulin resistance.

The squirrels, penguins, whales, fish, birds, they all do it. The hummingbird will run blood sugars up to 700; the liver becomes white from eating nectar, high fructose sugar, in one day.

Metabolic syndrome should be called the fat storage syndrome. That's why I wrote my last book called "The Golden Opportunity" to encourage providers to diagnose this increasing medical problem very early. I recommend health risk assessment and blood testing starting as a young child and then possibly we might avoid most of this plague.

Insulin resistance is a survival factor in animals, but it's killing us because we have lost the uricase enzyme and the ability to make vitamin C and they control the fat switch in the mitochondria, according to Dr. Richard Johnson, and I agree with that after reviewing the relevant medical literature.

Animals develop metabolic syndrome to survive. But food is plentiful for us and we don't need it. Very little evolutionary selection will occur among humans in the future because we're dying generally beyond the reproductive age and nature will not get panicked about it. But we are leading sickly lives, losing our memory and dying young of chronic diseases. Very little evolutionary selection will occur. Most people will be through the reproductive years before they die.

Obesity is not from gluttony and idleness, but because we've activated the same switch all animals use to increase fat stores. Industry is, of course, looking for the pill to affect the fat switch. Good luck fighting the survival mechanism of Mother Nature. I'd rather teach you how to eat correctly.

The cause of obesity is that we are eating too much and exercising too little, right? Culture, economics and behavior support that. Eating too much, because of fast food, cheap food, allows us to ingest massive amounts of calories. All-you-can-eat buffets, sugary drinks, high fructose corn syrup and lack of exercise on top of that.

The average child is exposed to 40,000 food advertisements a year, 72% for fast food.

Animals have a set point, we don't. Probably because we lack the ability to throw the fat switch off. The lack of uricase enzyme acquired in evolution is largely responsible.

Obesity is generally measured by the BMI, body mass index: Weight/kilogram divided by height in meters squared, 20-25 is normal, 25-30 is overweight, greater than 35 is obese, greater than 42 was morbidly obese.

The Obese are on Fire

THE FRUCTOSE PRESENT IN FRUITS, vegetables and high fructose drinks is part of the driver of our obesity epidemic, although just plain sugar, which is 50% fructose, probably is the main person at the wheel.

Let's face it: carrot cake has 50 grams of fructose.

One in 5 people in the Persian Gulf has type 2 diabetes, while 40% are obese, higher than in the United States. I bet you 70% or higher have "diabesity," the path to type 2 diabetes. Saudi Arabia and Kuwait are leading the way and are surrounded by countries that are also being invaded by this epidemic.

Thirty-5 million people in the Middle East and North Africa have type 2 diabetes -- 11% of the world has now come down with the disease. The situation is predicted to become much worse. It is predicted to grow to 68 million in the Middle East by 2035. Sub Sahara Africa is having great increases at this time.

I found out recently that the famous clinic, Lifestyle Institute in Arizona, which had reversed type 2 diabetes over a 3-week period for 30 years, has closed according to an operator I spoke to. They did follow-up studies and found very poor compliance in their former patients. Due to these poor long-term results, they decided to close. This has put an arrow through my heart, but it will not stop me and I will just redouble my efforts. After all, I am a doctor.

The good news is that this plague can be prevented, stopped and reversed. Let's get to work. 90 percent of type 2 diabetes can be stopped, reversed and prevented over just 4 to eight weeks. But, we need good follow up to make sure that we are inducing a permanent change. Low compliance rates are not going to work. Then again, most people can indeed be cured the majority of the time.

Dr. Mehmet Oz says, "Inflammation is the rusting of your arteries." Inflammation is a fire where you can't see the flames. It remains hidden for many years until you run some tests, and then it might be too late.

The Omega-6 invasion

CHOLESTEROL IS WHAT AMERICANS WORRY about the most. Cholesterol is a risk factor but does nothing proven to cause heart disease. Dr. Steven Sinatra wrote a book, a good read called "The Myth of Cholesterol."

We've known since 1975 fat thromboxanes, pro-inflammatories, like Omega-6 can kill.

In 1985 researchers from around the world came to a conference in Washington DC to examine claims that essential fatty acids, like Omega-3's and Omega-6's found in plant oils and people who eat fish confers special benefits and were good for your health.

The conference was paid for by the National Fishery Institute, Department of Commerce, and the National Institute of Health, with the goal of promoting consumption of fish and fish oil, which it did.

But it caused us actually to pay more attention to Omega-3's and Omega-6 consumption.

The scientist had begun to study the membranes of our 70 trillion body cells and their fatty acid composition.

The idea emerged that our Omega-6's in the diet were too high.

Dr. Dyerberg and Dr. Bang of Denmark studied the fat composition of the Eskimo diet. Their work eventually led to the discussion of the discovery of the essential fatty acids. The invention of gas liquid chromatography helped a great deal. The Eskimos as you remember were consuming a 60% high fat fish diet and had no evidence of vascular disease.

Participants came into the meeting thinking that eating fish was enough to give us large amounts of omega-3s but left the meeting that fish may not be enough to prevent the chronic diseases linked to a diet that was high in omega-6 fats.

People walk around with seemingly good health but are consuming a high meat diet rich in omega-6's. They tested the tissues to find that out. 78% of the people in the US had higher omega-6's, 50% in Italy and Greece, at 47% in Japan. That seems to correlate to the incidence in these countries.

Mortality from heart disease goes up in a linear fashion with the consumption of Omega-6's, the pro-inflammatory fatty acid.

The rates of deaths from heart disease was 50/hundred thousand in Japan, 90/hundred thousand in the Mediterranean, and 200/hundred thousand in the US. That's highly significant.

Where do the Omega-3's and 6's come from? All the greens including corn, wheat, Bogart, soybeans, vegetable oils are high in omega-6's. Omega-3s are found in fish, olive oil, and nuts.

There are many more Omega-6's in processed food. By adding a hydrogen atom to hydrogenated vegetable oils that increased the Omega-6's. Hydrogenation is a technique that was invented at the turn of the 19th century to turn vegetable oils into solid fat by limiting all the double bonds in its fatty acid chains. Margarine, for example, is a low cost alternative to lard and butter, despite partially hydrogenated oils.

Omega-3's and 6's, Alpha-linoleic acid are lost during hydrogenation.

Partially hydrogenated vegetable oils have more omega-3 than Omega-6. The detail of that science was not known until later. So it took a long time to spread this discovery around and have it reflected in what were eating.

The conference decided the diet was out of whack.

So it's the "evil twins" sugar and fructose and now the evil brother Omega-6 has arrived and that's why we are exploding and burning down our bodies.

Our agriculture, food processers, the government, FDA, USDA, AHA, and Ancel Keys are ganging up on us with bad advice.

The USDA has been keeping track of fat consumption ever since 1909 and they say Omega-6 consumption is steadily increasing. From 7 g/per day-225/grams per day.

Part of this was due to the recommendation to use more vegetable oils.

Saturated fat as a percentage of total fat consumption has actually fallen from 42 to 39%. This should have caused a decrease in the incidence of heart disease. But it hasn't. That's because fat is not the biggest part of the problem, sugar is. Mortality rate of heart disease has dropped some because of better medical treatment but not by the teaching of prevention.

The incidence of mortality from our disease actually has gone up with rising Omega-6's of which Israel consumes more per capita than any other country in the world, greater than 30 g daily. This is known as the Israeli paradox. But it's only paradox to those who don't distinguish between Omega-3's and 6's.

Israelis eat less animal fat and cholesterol and fewer calories than Americans, but have comparable rates of heart disease, obesity, diabetes and cancer. Israel may be regarded as a dietary experience of the effect of high Omega-6, polyunsaturated fats diet.

At the conference in 1985 the available food tables contained very few green vegetables. Spinach, leaks, kale, broccoli, actually have significant amounts of fats, mainly Omega-3's and more than they actually thought. After all the energy from the sun is picked up by α-Linolenic acid (ALA)

, It's in every leaf. Just think, ALA is in every leaf in the world. The roots of plants are full of Omega-6's; incidentally all plants are high in omega-3's, anti-inflammatories.

Linseed, flaxseed, are high in omega-3's, also the weed purslane is full of omega-3's.

Americans have a lot less omega-3's because they consume a lot more animal products.

The same pattern is in free-range grain fed beef, lamb, and pork and milk, as well as pond fed fish. It all depends on what the animals is eating. What they eat is what you eat. Free range or Cafo fed (concentrated animal feeding organizations).

ALA a is a fat that plants used in the membrane of the chloroplast, the fat that surrounds their complex machinery of photosynthesis enables plants to capture the photons of the sun and turns them into carbohydrate.

What's happening is that we are consuming, more seeds, and less leaves and then the Omega-6's are increasing and omega 3 are decreasing which is a major contributor to chronic disease. The change started since introduction of agriculture 10,000 years ago but is accelerated in the last hundred years. Extracting oils from seeds also has speeded up the process.

Fish has become important to human health as a source of omega-3's. Also, they have larger amounts of DHA, EPA, ALA, then animals. They consume mainly phytoplankton's, the most prevalent plant in the world. The oceans are not as healthy as they used to be either in that is of some concern. Fish eat algae, plankton and other fish.

The phytoplankton is the largest plant mass on the planet, it contributes the largest amount of ALA – the good fat.

Fish conceived in aquaculture farming have more grains in them. Therefore the fish you eat should be from the ocean. I always asked the waiter where the fish came from.

Dr. Simopolous was one of the first to compare the fats in wild animals and cultivated greens and Michael Crawford compared fats in domesticated animals. All of which led to the supplement food industry like omega-3 eggs.

Dr. Simopoulis work led to the underlying knowledge that most of our Omega-3's in the diet ultimately come from green leaves and most of Omega-6's come from seeds. Fish consumption counts but an overconsumption of seed oils and under consumption of green leaves lead to inflammatory state.

Our tissues are full of stored, troublesome, pro-inflammatory essential fatty acids. As Dr. Robert Lustig says, "We are not fit to eat."

Americans consume 11-16 g of Omega-6 per day and 1-2 g of ALA. Only 15% is converted to DHA our fast and essential fatty acid.

The Eskimos diet has been changing and not for the better. Dr. Dyerberg and Dr. Bang revisited the Eskimo villages and their eating the Western diet now. The Eskimos said, "We told you it was the fat that is healthy."

The explanation for the change in heart disease is that they consume large amounts of other fats that compete with the fat in fish and seal. Let's face it it's different fat. Much more Omega-6 fat.

Ralph Holman from Minnesota, the famous nutritionist, expresses, "Metabolism will happen whether we like it or not." Omega-6 will be converted to AA no matter how much omega-3 were eating because of a high consumption of vegetable oils, hydrogenated food products, pond fed fish, meat from concentrated animal feeding organizations. We are eating a pro-inflammatory diet on the average.

In other words you have to reduce you Omega-6 consumption if you want any benefit from the Omega-3's. Eat more omega 3 and less Omega-6 and avoid the evil twins sugar and fructose.

Since 1985 we pay much more attention to the essential fatty acids but it was also the beginning of the split and a large disconnect between scientists who study fats and the government and medical groups and industry that made the recommendations about what a healthy diet is.

As of 2005 the USDA dieter guidelines, the cornerstone of federal nutritional policy, did not distinguish between different families of essential fatty acids.

As of 2004 the American Heart Association did not distinguish between the family of fats, omega-3 and omega-6's. They said in 2004, "Polyunsaturated fats and monounsaturated fats are 2 unsaturated fats." The Institute of Medicine of the National Academy of Science recommended a 10/1-omega-6-omega-3 diet, which we know had a high degree of heart disease associated with it.

The Swedes recommended a 5/1-omega-6-omega-3, and the Japanese recommended 4/1-omega-6-omega-3 diet.

The government has been slow to act because of the amount of money involved. The edible oil industry is a very powerful lobby and the soybean and corn lobby were running the show through politics and lobbying money.

Cardiologist and the pharmaceutical industry didn't want us to change: business is business. Angioplasties pay a lot more and lobby money keeps politicians in office.

The scientists, government and AHA have dominated medical thinking and the new medicine was more difficult to understand by the public. To understand fat metabolism is not easy and complicated for the public. I've been trying. Reducing saturated fat has been around for 50 years.

Food labeling has helped, but is tricky to interpret. They did not make it easy for the public like they do in Europe. The food industry certainly had something to do with that with the lobby money. Decreasing omega-6 consumption is fine but you need to increase omega-3 consumption.

It may be little easier with supplements, eating a lot of fish, flax, omega-3 oil, and recommendations to increase fish consumption and greens. We're trying to put the fire out.

The complications of chronic disease are huge which occur because of high glucose, fructose and omega-6 consumption. Resulting in vascular disease, heart disease, strokes, type 2 diabetes, cancer, autoimmune disease. Next after were not all the same, some of us a more fire than others.. Your homocysteine level and CRP level may give you a clue.

Before the 1960s there were very few ways to distinguish the omega-3 and omega-6. The discovery photo spectroscopy in the early 1960s helped, that is mentioned previously. They used to all be grouped into polyunsaturated assets, "PUFA."

A researcher named Lawrence Rudl of Wake Forest University School of medicine found omega-3's low in animals with significant arteriosclerosis.

The" pacemaker theory" of leaky membranes hypothesis was eventually formulated by studying the membranes of cells extensively. This led to the study of metabolic rates. The rates of metabolic activity varied from animal to animal. Why? The protein in cell enzyme components was very similar in most cells of different animals. The total amount of fat in the cells was the same in most animals but the type of was not.

Saturated fat was high in slow animals. In the cell membranes, the fats of slow animals were full of saturated fat and high in omega-6.

A hummingbird was full of DHA, omega-3 and that is why they had very high speed wings. After eating you could see the fat through their skin, they needed it for energy and fast metabolism.

High DHA resulted in leaky membranes, and the DHA correlated better with metabolic rate.

Some described DHA as "molecular spring", that's where the action is. You couldn't be an astronaut or a pilot if you didn't have a high amount of DHA, a higher omega-3 diet. The brain is very sensitive to slight differences in fatty acids. The Japanese have high omega-3 in their body and a high pace of life. They're also the leanest.

Skeletal muscle is a major user of glucose in the body. The liver uses 20% of the sugar, brain 20%, and 60% estate cannot buy the muscles. The difference DHA content is different in humans, animals, races, the type of diet you eating.

The composition of your fatty acids has a strong influence on the binding of insulin to its receptors in humans as well as in rats. The implications for insulin resistance and development of diabetes is huge.

The research people have said that funding from NIH and the US Department of Agriculture is difficult to get for long-term studies of omega-3's and omega-6's. But we now know that glucose, fructose, and inflammatory omega-6's are the cause of most chronic diseases.

2 faces of sugar - Brain booster and brain buster

20% OF BLOOD GLUCOSE GOES to the brain, 20% to the liver and 60% to the muscles. So sugar is the preferred fuel. Brain cells and neurons metabolize sugar only, others can run on fat.

The brain is 2% of body weight but consumers 20% of the sugar.

Glucose is transported to the mitochondria our energy factories. Too little glucose headers memory but also too much sugar elevation impairs memory.

Our aging brain may need more glucose.

So we need sugar but high circulating levels of sugar and insulin result in degradation of memory and mental functioning, partially because of diabetes and pre diabetes.

The twin devils high insulin levels, and high sugar levels can be hazardous to your brain. High sugar and high insulin levels may cautery stiff, less elastic, and decreased blood flow to the brain.

Controlling blood sugar and insulin should be high priorities at all ages.

It has been proven that high sugar and diabetic children results in a decreased IQ.

Older diabetics are 3 times more apt to show significant signs of cognitive decline. This is been proven in mental tests.

High insulin levels may be detrimental to" synaptic activity" interfering with memory and brain activity. Especially the functioning of our synaptic activity.

There is a higher rate of dementia and Alzheimer's disease among type II diabetics. Some people call Alzheimer's disease type III diabetes.

Summaries searchers think brain cells are resistant to the transfer of sugar forebrain cell function in diabetics. Some disagree.

It is quite clear though the type II diabetics have memory problems and this is been proven. In my experience of neurology and neurosurgery for 44 years when reviewing CT scans and MRIs I consistently saw a lot of changes in the white matter of the brain, correlating the problems I was seeing, memory loss and strokes.

Some scientists believe some cases of Alzheimer's disease are clearly linked to diabetes. Autopsies done on diabetics reveal high rates of vascular disease, especially in the small vessels. The 300,000 miles of capillaries that we have resulting in retinopathy, neuropathy, advance heart and kidney disease.

High glycemic index foods lead to insulin resistance or pre diabetes.

With insulin resistance, inflammation of our extensive vascular system promotes hypertension, Ontario and atherosclerosis.

High blood sugars can lead to age associated and products, the combination of protein and sugar called Age's that can be deposited all over our body it is the main cause of advanced aging, arteriosclerosis, memory loss, unto sclerosis and makes us look old. It causes age-related damage known as glycation.

The point is to avoid excessive glucose, fructose and omega-6's in the body because the increase information, glycation and other cause of the chronic fire in our body.

Glycation is like what happens to a chicken when you roasted. The skin gets browned and Rusty. Basically we are cooking slowly over a lifetime-we are simmering.

Oxygen free radicals, which occur from too much metabolic activity, it eating too many calories, have the same effect and part of the inflammatory process.

In Israel research has revealed that they may be eating too much fructose to account for the hide incidents of vascular disease. Heck, fructose is what we've been talking about.

The bottom line is high blood sugar levels of glucose, fructose, a smile as I consumption of omega-6 fatty acids through the eating of vegetable oils, nonorganic raised animals and pond fish are kindling the fire in our body the brain was not designed to accommodate such considerable overloads of modern sugary foods and is reacting to them.

Sitting disease

WHOEVER HEARD OF THAT DISEASE? Really they speak with anyone who knows what it is.

Just to shock you, it is now considered to have more importance on your health than smoking. Wow!

To get right down to it, we know most of us a sitting a lot more, sometimes for the eight hours a day. A scientific study proved that sitting for 4-5 hours daily without movement is worse than the effects of smoking on your health.

Interestingly, diet and sitting for 4 to 5 hours has been found to be worse than smoking effect on your health. As said by Dr. David Katz in his excellent book "Disease Proof," 80% of our chronic diseases can be prevented through good health habits and lifestyle. So there is room for optimism if we act.

The biological need to walk or exercise is great effect on our genes through epigenetics. Yes, we can temporarily a generation or 2, affect our genetic structure, good or bad, by our lifestyle and health habits.

Let's have a look at our daily calorie burn.

About 60% is determined by Howard B and R, basic metabolic rate, the bigger you are the higher the rate.

10% of calories are used up as is the thermic effect of food-digestion. Another 5% or so can be used up by regular exercise, but, believe it or not, only 3.5% of the people exercise regulates.

That has been scientifically study. We thought it was 10 to 15% but detailed studies don't support that.

The other 30% is called "neat activity," no exercise activity thermogenics. That includes our daily routine activities of work, walking the dog, cooking and doing the dishes, using the stairs instead of the elevator etc. it's that 30% that we can work out to increase calorie burn.

Using the stairs instead of the elevator, parking a car further than the usual place, walking once around the food market before shopping, dancing at home, standing up when you're on the phone, using a treadmill when using the computer. The hardest other things you do to increase your calorie burn during the day.

Increasing your calorie burn too many calories a day results in the 20 pound weight loss in one year, 300 cal a day would result in the 30 pound weight loss in the year, if you don't change anything else. Obviously if you watched it which are eating the weight loss will be a great deal more. Standing instead of sitting increases the calorie burn times 3.

There is a whole new of scientific studies looking at inactivity to promote good health. The science of prolonged sitting is very interesting. You actually have neat cells in your body that don't respond to rigorous exercise but to gentle muscle contractions.

Increasing your neat activity is one of the best things you can do for your health, especially your heart. It starts at the cellular level.

Your capillaries, the tiny blood vessels that deliver oxygen and nutrients rich blood into your tissues throughout the body aligned with special cells called endothelial cells that assist the flow of blood. These cells contain an enzyme called protein lipase-LPL. Its job is to break down fat molecules, triglycerides.

These blood fats cause of most of heart disease. When you're sitting for a few hours these enzymes switch off. Sitting for the whole day their activity level is reduced 50%.

Eat a high-fat meal after sitting all day you can watch your blood fats skyrocket 180%.

The mere act of getting out of your chair is all it takes to break out of the hibernation mode.

Vigorous activity only increases your weight muscle fiber-the fast switch muscle.

That is why walking and increasing your neat activity every single day is so most important.

A constellation of risk factors for heart disease, diabetes, strokes, cancer, hypertension and autoimmune disease. Among females the rest of metabolic syndrome increased 26% for every hour they spend watching TV.

Every 30 minutes spent on increasing need activity reduce the risk and provided protection. A study done at Harvard proved walking provided the most protective exercise against heart disease.

Sitting disease makes a good luncheon presentation at work, I've done it many times.

The Motivation of Placebo and Nocebo

PLACEBO MEANS TO PLEASE, NOCEBO means to harm. A pill, a doctor, and occasionally even a procedure can result in healing if we believe that it will. That's the power of the placebo. The placebo effect can be between 30 to 70%. It depends on our faith in that medication, it causes chemical changes in our body and brain and we become well. It's been known about for thousands of years.

So a doctor, a medication and yes, even an operation, which found nothing, can motivate us toward wellness, It's all over the medical literature and in my personal experience in over 40 years of medical practice. The reason I always wear fancy clothes in my office is because it produces confidence in my patients. The patient believes I can get them well. Their chemistry responds and motivates them to get well.

A healthcare provider, overweight, out of shape will have difficulty motivating the patient through the placebo effect. The placebo costs little and is very cheap. And a loving healthcare provider, the occasional hug, the smile, and friendly conversation, beginning with. "What's going on in your life?" can heal the patient.

Recently, I was treating the owner of a company with 35 employees for severe sciatica. I found nothing on the MRI scan, and did not recommend surgery. I tried every measure possible, but he just did not get better. One day he came to me and said, if I did nothing to help him, he would have to close his small factory on Monday and put 35 people out of work. This made the situation even more serious; 35 people could lose their job. I told him I could explore the nerve that I thought was involved with this pain and see if he had a hidden ruptured disk. I operated on him and found nothing. Trying to be a healer, not trying to be his deceitful, I told him I took some pressure off the nerve by removing some arthritic bone, and gave a lot more room to the nerve. The following day, all this pain was gone, and he was back at work on Monday, and so were 35 other people. I think it was the placebo effect of the operation. That can happen. I am sure that surgeons who generally over operate (believe me there are plenty of them) take full of vantage of that. And that patients many times are better for a few months through the placebo effect. You can see a placebo can be motivating in itself. Because of your belief in what is done, or the pill or the health-care provider, faith causes chemical changes in the body and can motivate you to wellness.

The nocebo can motivate you toward unnecessary procedures. The healthcare provider takes advantage of modern technology, like CT scans, MRIs, scoping procedures and angiograms to impress you that the changes on the studies are related to your complaints, when many times they are not, to do a procedure on you. I see this a lot in back surgery, gallbladder surgery, hysterectomies, cosmetic surgery and an occasional heart operation. I have personally experienced that many times in my 40 years of practicing surgery. In essence, the nocebo, the negative speak, is used to promote a procedure. They hand you the CT, MRI, angiographic report, and you carry it around with you convincing you of the seriousness of your problem, when in reality it may not mean very much. That makes it a lot easier for the provider to talk you into something. That's why I called the "nocebo" the evil twin. It can motivate you toward an unnecessary operation or procedure. I've written a book called "**Nocebo - Placebo's Evil Twin**." You might enjoy reading it and it may save you an unnecessary procedure. The book can be found on my website www.kachmannmindbody.com.

Our Frontal Lobe Is in Charge and Motivates Us

ONE WAY OR ANOTHER, WE are the ones who will make the decision on what to eat. We are the authors of our own health. We are the driver of that tank that is involved with this war of eating.

Women have more eating problems than men because they are in charge more of the meal preparation, buying the food, and a constant barrage from the media and magazines about body size.

Can you imagine buying food for a husband, yourself, and the children who all have different appetites and food preferences, and she is trying to control the situation. The husband may have the "inflexible palate syndrome" and just will not change what he eats in spite of being a diabetic or heart patient. The husband says, "I can't possibly live without eating meat every day." The children are screaming out for sugary, fatty and salty foods.

I would say with children it's a bit easier, because they will get hungry and you are buying the food. If there is a problem and your children are overweight, have an honest look at them. Don't deny the picture, bring in changes slowly, and they may not notice it. Their tastes buds will change. I slowly introduced a lot of vegetarian food at the doctors' lounge in the hospital. Frankly, they did not notice it and the food looks great now.

The dietitian is a friend of mine. Next week she's bringing in edamame on a regular basis. Sooner or later, the children's tastes buds will change. Educate them about school food, to read labels, to avoid sugary drinks. The husband could be more of a problem. He may need to be educated about healthy food. Believe me, in my 45 years of being a physician; Americans in general eat the mad, toxic, sad foods, all fat, sugar, and salt. The killer triad of Americans.

Limiting your own or family members food intake is like a starvation diet; it will not work and will result in over eating and snacking. When preparing food yourself on a daily basis. It makes it a lot more difficult, and quite easy to feed your own psychology with food. The food that causes the flow of dopamine is in your hand, a very tempting situation. Besides, you may be hungry. You look at food every day, making the meals and testing your self-control daily and sometimes multiple times a day. It is difficult for many. Family members may use food to control each other socially. One never eats; another over eats. One is perfect, and another is out of control. Being overweight, people think you're out of control, that you have emotional problems. Thinness is considered being in control, but many times it is not.

Society looks at people with a normal weight as being in control of their lives. Social stigma is related to body size.

Eating control was thought to be the solution to obesity, when the answer to me is much more the type of food you are eating. Control will follow that if you're eating the correct food. If you are eating a high nutrient dense food pattern, in general, you do not need to watch even your portions. Most of the time, it is difficult for us to have perfect control of our eating habits. I say, "food selection" should lead the way to good health and proper weight.

Over-controlling behavior with food is a central problem with eating disorders, anorexia and bulimia.

You'll get some families, like I saw last week, gathered around the table at a Japanese restaurant, where I clearly saw them all, twenty feet in front of me, from 3-year-olds to 80-year-olds, about 10 of them, all seriously overweight. Children with puffy cheeks, adults with bellies hanging down, men and women. It was a sad sight. I would say odds are they a totally blind to their situation. Just like an anorexic.

How did this happen? Genetics accounts for only 20%. Probably they're like the anorexic, and many overweight people, they don't see it in themselves. You do not see the potential health problems, and that is frankly all I'm talking about. I don't care about the cosmetics; many of these people are beautiful. I passionately care about their future of diabetes, heart disease and strokes, arthritis, dementia and cancer. Their psychiatric needs and eating behavior probably are the same throughout the family; the anxiety and probably the lack of serotonin to feel good are about the same. Instead of a tranquilizer, they are using food to feel good. They have a similar way of cooking, same type of food, most likely lack of proper eating education. I would bet 2 or 3 already have diabetes, maybe one of them even as a teenager. I would bet everything I own that the 2 or 3 diabetics do not know that their type 2 diabetes is curable by getting down to a normal weight.

Food preferences are transmitted within the family from parent to child. Pleasurable fatty food, and sugary food, chemically decreases anxiety, increases love. It's the womb, that caves, and escape from life's problems. The poor have this need, of course, more commonly. That is the reason they have a much higher rate of overweight and obesity. It's their only daily pleasure, many times. There is much more obesity in the economically distressed. Food is also used among family members to distribute power, rewards, and to control behavior. Eating behavior is used many times among family members to assume power and control.

Eating behavior can keep the family together: the hell with the rest of the world, this is us! An individual's thoughts and beliefs and attitudes greatly affect what they eat. Many people justify their food choices with incorrect information they obtain from some ineffective diet book. Many of the diet books are complete frauds. Individuals have a range of beliefs about the meaning of food system, body size and shape. Many believe diets are all or nothing and give up too easily.

Food deprivation will lead to overeating. High-protein diets don't work. Starving yourself of carbohydrates will sooner or later lead to overeating. Negative beliefs about obesity may motivate some people to a normal weight—I don't want to look this way—and they become motivated to change. It's a complex psychological situation between the pleasure of eating and subsequent guilt.

As we know, women are the main providers of food in the family. Gender is central to many of the conflicts surrounding food. Eighty percent of the clients in my eating classes are female. There are a number of reasons for that. They also choose education about proper eating more commonly. Men don't want to give up that steak and would rather exercise. Women are treated differently in the media. You have to be thin to be on TV, although we have witnessed the yo-yo diets of Oprah. I suspect that situation is all about psychology. Women show more body dissatisfaction than men, and also body size is more important to women's self-esteem.

Most of the anorexics and bulimics are women. Abdominal fat is more dangerous, and men have more of that; female fat is usually around the buttocks and thighs.

Food choice is affected by social norms. Certain ethnic groups make better or worse, food choices. The famous China study by Dr. Colin Campbell, where they studied Chinese people and related eating patterns. In other cultures, overweight and obesity is rampant in more than 50% of the people, and those cultures have diabetes and its consequences. Family and cultural norms affect our image of ourselves. Certain ethnic groups accept obesity.

Dieting, not food selection is a media choice to lose weight. Which sells diet books, but they usually don't work. They're not concerned since they already made the money.

Social norms of attractiveness, contribute to the discrimination and stereotypes of being overweight and obese. Peer influence and social support can be used to modify eating behavior in the overweight. And this is a socially desirable state, which can lead to eating disorders. The psychological effects of the chemicals of food—dopamine, serotonin, endorphins, and beta-endorphin—probably are the great drivers of food choices and habits.

The individual, the family, the group, have great effects on the food choices that we make. Some ethnic groups think cheese is everything, although, mind you, it's 80% fat.

We have to eat every day, so the cue is there continuously, lack of serotonin cries out for relief. It will take a combination of stress relief, exercise and food choice that will lead to proper eating habits and good health. You are the author of your health! Fat, sugar and salt have the nasty chemicals that lead to being overweight and obese. Good luck in your choices.

Authority

READING A BOOK, ATTENDING A lecture, listening to educational CDs, talking to an expert in the field, M.D., or Ph.D. are all ways that can motivate us. There is a genetic tendency in us to listen and follow the recommendations of an authority figure.

We have a deep-seated sense of duty to authority. This has been studied scientifically. It is the extreme willingness of adults to go to almost any lengths on the command of an authority that constitutes the chief findings of a scientific study. Doesn't that make you wonder about what happened in Germany in the '30s and '40s? Authority was obeyed without question at that time in history, which led to war and the Holocaust.

So "authority" can lead to good, improving your life, health job, and relationships, but also to an extreme. As we see in terroristic acts today, largely related to extreme positions in religion, faith, brainwashing, and to the point of suicide in the name of a cause. So the authority you pick and believe in is critical.

The appearance of authority can be enough. We are often vulnerable to the symbols of authority. Just the symbol of M.D., Ph.D., or a uniform increases their believability, and we are more likely to obey them. Several symbols can reliably trigger our compliance in the absence of any clear knowledge of that authority person. Con artists drape themselves with the symbols of authority. They drive up in a fancy car, fancy clothes, college degrees they don't have and are smooth talkers. They know they are adorned by the principal of authority compliance on our part.

There's no question the size of the authority figure can make a difference. It's in our genetic code. Look at animal behavior, who's in charge of their tribe? The big guy.

In my own experience, as soon as I could afford them. I've always dressed in a nice suit, ties and shoes and drove a fancy car. Believe me, it improved my credibility and ability to motivate my patients to wellness. I'm a surgeon, but I tell you 2 thirds of my time I spend talking to patients, trying to get them to motivate toward wellness, weight loss, stress reduction, and exercise. There's no question, I spend 2 thirds of my time teaching patients. It thrills me to know that I can get all the patients well with the word and not the knife. If I can motivate them it will work.

We have a click-whir type of responding and people will take advantage of it. We stop thinking when an authority figure talks to us. But the good part is, if this is their authority, it causes us to change our behavior, quickly and motivate toward wellness. Maybe buying the CD or DVD of an authority you like can reinforce your daily and result in long-term improvement of your health, physically and mentally.

The white coat of a physician, or a nice suit is very significant. More authority than the out-of-shape, poorly dressed, unloving healthcare provider. Your doctor needs to be a placebo; you need to believe in his healing power. If the healthcare provider is not following his recommendations to you, I suspect he will not be a good motivator for you.

People calmly ask me, do I follow the recommendations of my book, "The Secret of the Nondiet," which I teach? You can is look at me and it's quite obvious that I do. It's motivating to the people I'm speaking to. If I weighed 230 pounds, you think they would listen to me? It would not be motivating.

If the authority figure drives a fancy car, it can have an effect on his authority, pro or con. We need to have a heightened awareness of the authenticity of the provider were listening to. Is the authority sincere, honest, and does he have your best interests at heart? Don't follow the authority to the grave. You know from reading the newspaper that that happens periodically. The Germans followed a powerful figure to the Holocaust. Is the authority truly an expert? Are his degrees real?

There is a genetic component in our mind and strong pressure from society to comply with requests of authority. The strength of this tendency to obey legitimizes the authority. It comes from systematic social practices designed and instilled in us from childhood. It implies obedience, constitutes correct conduct, right or wrong. It can lead to the good and the bad. Sometimes we respond to authority automatically. It is much more likely to happen when the authority has all the symbols, the degrees, the uniform, the stature, the fancy car, the supporting people and perhaps even CDs, DVDs and books. We accord such a person more deference and obedience upon the first encounter. You have to separate faith from facts. That can be very difficult.

Visualization

VISUALIZATION IS THE LANGUAGE OF the subconscious mind; in essence, it is how we speak to the brain.

If we create an image of what we would like to achieve, it is more likely to happen. Your brain will not be able to differentiate between what is real and what is not when you speak to it in pictures and images.

It can be very motivating and brings your thoughts into action. The human body contains about 70 trillion cells, and by creating images you are motivating these cells into action.

How does visualization work? Our bodies in the universe are essentially composed of energy. A thought is a quick and mobile force of energy. When we create or accomplish something, we always do it first by using our thought process. Thinking precedes action. Any image creates energy, and having an idea, picture, or thought tends to attract and create that energy form into reality.

We are always attracting the energy of life - whatever we think about the most, believe in the most, or are able to visualize most vividly.

When you visualize your goal, it is much more likely to happen because the act of creating images, or visualization, immobilizes and motivates your 70 trillion plus body cells into action.

Visualization works best after a period of meditation and deep breathing. While sitting in the yoga position or sitting in a chair, take about 10 to 20 deep abdominal breaths and create a picture over your goal. Use all of your senses - smells, feelings, tastes, sounds, and detailed pictures. Do it frequently. If you are visualizing weight loss, picture yourself on the beach during the morning sunrise, wearing great workout clothes, ready to go. Begin your stretch while you smell the ocean air, hear the waves, and feel the warmth of the sun energizing your body. Start your stretching and visualize yourself taking off on a beautiful morning run down the shore. Or imagine that new car, house, or career. You may even imagine doing missionary work and the great feeling it gives you.

When you have the image in your mind, make some affirmative statements to yourself, silently or out loud. "I'm going to lose those 30 pounds; I will have that great job; I will stop smoking; I will stop drinking; I will stop taking so many medications; I will cure my Type 2 Diabetes with proper eating." There are no limits to what you accomplish through the use of imagery and visualization!

The more frequently you do this, and the more detail you give to using your 5 senses, the most likely you are to achieve your goal. Affirmative statements are very motivating.

Learn to use meditation or deep breathing first so that you are in a relaxed state, this de-stresses your body and you will see the images more clearly. And, you are more likely to achieve your goal as you relax each muscle in your body. Count backwards from 20 – this is a mantra that will lead you into a meditative state. Meditation and visualization will relax you and renew your spirit and can be used during anytime of the day.

Imagery is a powerful and mysterious force in human nature that is able to bring about dramatic improvement in our lives. It is a kind of mental engineering that works best when supported by meditation, and especially strong religious faith. It is not difficult to practice and anyone can do it. It has caught the attention of doctors, psychologists, and "thinkers" everywhere. The word imagine is derived from imagination. Imagery, utilizing the feeling of mental pictures or images, is based on the principle that there is a deep tendency in human nature to become precisely like that which we imagine ourselves to be. An image formed and held tenaciously in the conscious mind passes the present state by use of a mental osmosis and travels into the unconscious mind. Once accepted firmly in the unconscious state, the individual strongly tends to grasp it, and it then becomes part of the individual. The imagery effect on thought and performance is so powerful that a long held vision of an objective or goal could become determinative.

Imaging is positive thinking. Carry this state one step further, and you could say that imaging is a laser beam of the imagination, a shaft of mental energy, in which the desired goal or outcome is pictured so vividly by the conscious mind that the unconscious mind accepts it and is activated by it. This release is so powerful in total force that it can bring about astonishing changes in the life of the person who is doing the imaging.

Let me give you some examples. Jim Thorpe, a famous Olympic athlete, while traveling by boat to Europe never practiced with the athletes on the ship. He never stretched, lifted weights, or jogged. Instead, he sat in the corner, using imagery, about every Olympic event he was to participate in. And, he won almost every track event! He had the used the power of imagery. My racecar friend, John Burton, who I play tennis with in Florida, once told me a story. Many of the famous racecar drivers imagine the event the night before, using imagery to successfully carry out their goals. Additionally, during the Vietnam War, an imprisoned sergeant, Sergeant Gordon, visualized playing 18 holes of golf every day for 7 years. When he was released from prison, during his first game in the United States he shot the best score of his life! That's the power of visualization. I always visualize my serve while playing tennis. And other athletes use this power all the time also. In sports, great athletes visualize what they wish to do, practice the living daylights out of it, and then they don't think when they play the sport, it has now become automatic.

There are 4 basic steps for effective visualization: to set your goal by tweaking a clear idea or picture, enhance this goal by using the 5 senses, focus on the goal often, and give yourself positive energy with affirmations of achieving this goal.

For many people, "affirmations" are most powerful and inspiring when they include references to a spiritual source. There are 3 elements within you that determine how to successfully create what will work for you in any given situation: desire, belief, and acceptance. These define your intention. Your spiritual source is a supply of infinite love, wisdom, and energy in the universe. Continue to practice your relaxation, visualization and affirmations daily.

<u>Healing</u>

Conscious creative visualization is a process of creating positive thoughts and images to communicate with our bodies - to remove our thoughts out of a place of negativity to a place of positivity, and to replace constrictive and what may be literally sickening thoughts with positive energy.

One can also use visualization and imaging to treat cancer. Dr. Carl Simington published a great book called *Getting Well Again*. In this book, he describes great visualization techniques to destroy cancer cells. If cancer is your problem this is a great book to read. It has helped a lot of cancer patients. Imaging can also be used to help your pain problems. As a neurosurgeon, I have had a lot of experience with this and it can be very helpful.

The anticipatory power of the imagination has been utilized in many sports, and scientific research has established its effectiveness for athletes. This research shows that by picturing the successful completion of moves they want to make, athletes can improve their performance - especially if the mental picture is accompanied with physical practice. Good athletes have physical and mental self-control. Jack Nicklaus, author of *Golf My Way*, claimed that hitting a good shot depends 10% on swing mechanics, 40% on set up and stance, and 50% on his mental picture. In his book he describes how to visualize a shot before he makes it; he describes it like making a very colorful movie. He never hit the shot, even in practice, without having a very sharp and focused picture of it in his head. First, he sees the ball, nice and white and sitting up high on the bright green grass. Then the scene quickly changes, and he sees the ball getting to where he wants it - its path, its trajectory and shape, even its behavior on the landing. Just make your movie that shows a perfect shot.

Imagery and healing is probably best known for its direct effects on your own physiology. Through imagery, you can stimulate changes in many bodily functions usually considered inaccessible by a conscious influence. Imagery is a natural language of a major part of our nervous system. It has been shown that the 2 sides of the human brain think in very different ways. They are simultaneously capable of independent thought. The left and right sides of the brain are different - the right side of the brain speaks in images; the left side of brain speaks more in terms of language and numbers. This essential difference between the 2 brains is a relatively new way of thinking. The left-brain processes information sequentially, while the right brain processes it simultaneously and specifically.

Imagery in Everyday Life

Imagery has been presented as a powerful device to achieve major goals and objectives. Use it everyday. It can be used to smooth out the minor wrinkles of living. Many famous inventions were produced by the use of imagery. Imagery has its own formula: the goal, purpose, prayer activity, thoughtful planning, innovative thinking, organization, hard work, and always holding the image of success firmly in mind. If this process is faithfully carried out, the desired results will be achieved, despite any and all difficulties or setbacks.

The Best of Dr. Rudy's Motivation Principles

"THE RUDY IN YOU" IS a great book about motivation to success in sports by Rudy Ruetigger. You may have seen the movie, which was about building teamwork, fair play and sportsmanship.

But my name is Rudy too. A lot of the principles laid down by Notre Dame's Rudy are actually what I teach to motivate success and wellness. Of the 40 or so most powerful motivators, I would like to pick the top 10 to my way of thinking.

Before I do that, I would like to tell you my story of my interest in motivation. Recently, I was the guest speaker at a National Chiropractic Association meeting. I gave my talk on reversing type 2 diabetes by eating a proper diet, and a very nice chiropractic doctor stood up and said, "Thank you. The information is great, but how do I motivate my patient to follow it?" I think that's a very fair question, and I decided to read a lot about it and write a book about it, as this information has only limited value if people don't use it to become well.

Why does Dr. Rudy (myself) have such a great interest in the teaching of wellness? For one, all my life I've had a great interest in playing sports of all types. I was not a natural athlete at anything. As a matter of fact, in high school I used to have to try to gain weight. In grade school and high school, I always tried to join a sports team, all the sports. I lived in New York City and played at Central Park every day, handball, tennis, and baseball. I tried very hard to become good at the sports but my ability was limited let's say at best, a little bit above average. My father had no interest in sports. He worked in his delicatessen day and night. Only through a lot of practice, did I get good enough to make the baseball team, basketball team, and, yes, even the football team. I had a lot of help, as it was a small school. I weighed only 135 pounds, but playing sports certainly was a good step to wellness. I was not an overweight teenager. My parents consistently ate the wrong deli food, fat, sugary and salty food. They were both overweight.

The teaching of exercise and nutrition was not part of medical school, and it barely is now. I was at my 45th medical school reunion recently and they said, does anyone have any questions? There were 3 female medical students at luncheon and I asked them how much they had learned about nutrition and wellness. All 3 said, very little. That was a very sad day for me, and it still has not changed.

After I started my practice and looked closely at my patients' medical problems, remember I'm a neurosurgeon; I developed a sense early in my practice that the majority of illnesses and diseases I was looking at were self-inflicted. Stress, lack of exercise, and what the patients were eating was a cause of 50 to 80% of what I was treating. Many were type 2 diabetics from being overweight. That could be simply corrected by being the proper weight. Then I found a book, *How to Live 365 Days a Year*, by Dr. Schindler. I handed out about 5,000 copies free to my patients. They took about $3,000 off my quarterly bonuses to pay for it by my corporation. And I was happy to do it. A lot of patients get well without injections, medications or surgery. I felt like I was a doctor doing what was right. After all, the word physician means teacher. We are not graduating teachers from the medical school.

Eventually I read everything I could get my hands on about wellness and found out that, frankly, it's all interrelated and my knowledge base grew tremendously. My motivation to teach this on a wider scale flew off the charts. I don't seem to be able to keep quiet about it, no matter where I go. I now have a wellness center with a yoga studio. We teach proper eating, exercise, individual and group training, meditation, stress reduction, dancing and many other programs. My website is www.KachmannMindBody.com. By December I will probably have 10 published books, all in every aspect of wellness. I formed the Mind-Body Index, a list of illnesses caused partially or totally by the mind, usually stress. I made about 20 CDs and DVDs, one-hour lectures on the effects of the aspect of the mind on the human body, about stress, cancer, exercise, proper eating, the nocebo effect, etc. I give at least 30 lectures a year on wellness and have a one-hour weekly TV show about wellness that attracts a large audience.

Clearly, it was a love of teaching the patient how to get well without having to give him dangerous medications or doing surgery that inspired me. Really, it's about the love for the patient, the ability to make them well in the safest manner, reducing the amount of illnesses and diseases that they have and increasing their longevity.

My Top 10 Motivators
- Food—what we eat
- Life changing events
- Visualization and imaging
- Commitment
- Power of positive thinking

- Mind-body connection
- The will to live
- Meditation
- Yoga and chi-gung
- Purpose

We all have different things that motivate us. Take a moment to write down 10 things that motivate you the most below.

1 _____

2 _____

3 _____

4 _____

5 _____

6 _____

7 _____

8 _____

9 _____

10 _____

Motivation and Breathing

MANY BREATHING TECHNIQUES LEAD TO wellness. The ancient Chinese, the Tao and the Hindu-yoga traditions, use breathing techniques extensively to achieve a quiet state of mind-mindfulness. That leads to good health and stress reduction.

The Buddha gives simple instructions that form the basis for breath meditation. The meditator assumes the Lotus position, "cross-legged posture." The only time that mindfulness can happen is in the present moment; if you think you know the past that is memory. Mindfulness is unbiased. It is not for or against anything. When you focus on the breath for a few moments, thinking calms itself. Therefore, you could be doing anything, walking, combing your hair, doing the dishes, if you are concentrating on your breath, this will lead to mindfulness. It's meditation.

When we focus on the breath, we are focusing on the life force. Life begins with the first breath and will end after our last. To contemplate breathing is to contemplate life itself. Ancient India had a tremendous respect for the breath, a deep understanding of its powerful effect on the body and mind. In fact, all of the Indian spiritual sciences had some form of pranayama, which is usually translated "breath control." Most forms of pranayama, yogic breathing, involve controlling the breath. The quality of the breathing does improve; it becomes fuller, freer and calmer, with consequences both physical and psychological. We're all breathing. We need to be aware of the simple sensation, the in breath and the out breath. We note that a deep breath relaxes the body and figure that an accomplished meditator will be breathing deeply all the time, period. If we allow the breath to unfold naturally, without tampering with it, in time we may be able to do that with other aspects of our experience, we might learn to let the feelings be, let the mind be. Using meditation in its extreme form allows you to develop a Zen mind. The ultimate goal, the Zen mind is not easy to achieve and takes time to develop.

The breath is an ideal vehicle for teaching Buddhism in the West. It is not religion. It's a way of being. A mindful way of life that leads to wellness.

For some people breathing it isn't a terribly pleasant process. A lifetime of faulty breathing, often accompanied by emotional blockages, has made the breath an unattractive object of attention. You need to develop a certain devotion to your meditation, like counting to 10, or repeating the same word to quiet the mind, in combination with the breathing techniques. Pick a time of day in a quiet place; it could be anywhere. You can meditate sitting at the stoplight, or cleaning the toilet.

An excellent way to relax is to concentrate on the breath when taking a walk. It's meditative and leads to healing of the stressful mind. At the beginning and at the end of a walk, stand and breathe mindfully for a few moments. Pay attention to every aspect of breathing, the nose, the lungs, the diaphragm and the abdomen. Breathe like a baby, so the belly hangs out when you breathe in deeply. Pay attention to every part of your body and your surroundings—its meditation. St. Francis of Assisi said, "It is no use walking anywhere to preach unless our walking is our preaching." There are 5 rewards for one who practices walking meditation: you can endure traveling by foot, you can endure exertion, you become free from disease, whatever you have eaten and drunk becomes well digested, and the concentration you win while doing walking meditation lasts a long time. It's this concentration, and the joy of walking in such a state that is the primary reward and a state of wellness is close behind.

Sometimes the breath is very fine, like silk or satin; it enters and exits freely. And other times it is coarse, more like burlap, and fights it's way in and out. Sometimes the breath is so deep in its root that it affects the whole body, relaxing it profoundly. As you pay attention to breathing, the quality of the breathing changes, perhaps because thinking is diminished. The breath becomes deeper, you find it more enjoyable, and the body starts to reap the fruits of that, to become more relaxed.

It just reflects the power of mindfulness. If your mind becomes angry, all worried, your heart starts to race, your body grows tense. But if you can just be with the breath for while, not suppressing the emotion, agreeing with it, all changes. The mind becomes calm. As the breath goes, so goes the body. The first law of Buddhism is that everything is constantly changing. So your breathing technique can change from time to time. Breathing leaves all the troubles behind, all the preoccupations, worries, plans, doubts, fears, all the stuff that makes up the mind. Especially in the modern world, where everybody is so impressed with variety and complexity, so desperate to be entertained, it is a relief to settle into the simple repetitive act. The opportunity we have of staying with the breathing, consciously coming back to it, is a chance to do one simple, ordinary thing well. Entry into the spirit of repetition can be a powerful lesson in simplicity, which is desperately needed in the modern world. Many people come to meditation expecting some complex practice leading to an ordinary experience. They can't believe they're just supposed to sit there and watch the breath. We begin to see how useful the skill is in other aspects of our lives. The constant repetition of going back to the breath has real value. In some ways this entire practice is everything the Buddha said, is concerned with having an infinite respect for life. The practice of breathing and meditation constantly reminds us that everything is worthy of attention. To be mindful of anything is an act of generosity. You are giving it life by allowing it into your world. But the greatest benefit is that you respect for your own life.

The breath is a vital conditioner of the body. The body, mind, and breath become one, and you are able to sit for a long time without pain or discomfort. It's important to emphasize that this process unfolds in different ways for different people, that it generally takes place over a long period of time, that for all, or most, of us it is the fruit of a great deal of sitting. It will cause us, though, to pay much more attention to what we are doing and get rid of destructive behaviors like overeating, lack of exercise, smoking, drinking and using drugs. All of the Buddha's teaching, it has been said, can be reduced to one, under no circumstances attach to anything as me or mine. It isn't that we shouldn't experience rapture or happiness, but that we have to be careful not to attach anything to them.

A huge amount of fear, anxiety, apprehension, is stimulated by thought itself. That is what you are trying to avoid by paying attention to the breath and developing relaxing mindfulness. A usual reaction to fear is to create a battlefield. Our fear is that war, with our tremendous yearning to be free from it, and the state of battle is the mind and the body in which the process is taking place. We tie ourselves into knots, turn ourselves inside out, fighting that battle. The attitude of practice is to open the process up, to see that it's all part of us, the fear, the yearning to be free of it, the mind and the body, the mindfulness observing them, the conscious breathing that nurtures the mindfulness. We sit there with all of that, all one thing. Then one day it comes up; our attention meets it, becomes one with it, allows it to blossom, which is what the fear wanted all along, and then you can get rid of it. It is when we prevent the blossoming of fear by ignoring its presence that fear hangs around, drags us down, because we spend so much energy holding it off. Even in the blossom, life has its parts. That way, you have all the energy you would have used escaping it to combat it. We also have the energy of the fear itself. It is a great gain in energy when we let things happen. The ground of fearlessness is fear. In order to become fearless, you have to stand in the middle of your fear. We shouldn't trust any fearlessness that doesn't have that as its basis. The beginning of that is to see your fear and admit to it. You acknowledge that you are afraid, and then have the immense courage and humility to study it. It can be the beginning of the end of it. In other words, make a plan to get rid of it. Don't try to suppress it.

Mindfulness and breathing techniques are the road to freedom of the mind.

The process of breathing shows us a way to let go of the old and be open to the new. The process of reading is a living metaphor for understanding how to expand our narrow sense of ourselves and to be present to the healing energies that are both in and around us. Some people say that the diaphragm is the" spiritual muscle". It lies at the foundation of healthy breathing. Shaped like a large dome, the diaphragm functions as both the floor of the chest cavity and the ceiling, all the abdominal cavity. When we inhale, the diaphragm normally contracts. This pump-like motion creates a partial vacuum, which as you know, draws air into the lungs. When we inhale fully, the diaphragm can double or even triple its range of movement and massage the stomach, liver, pancreas, intestines, and kidneys, promoting intestinal movement, blood and lymph flow, and the absorption of nutrients. The work of breathing starts with sensing the inner atmosphere of our organism, the basic emotional stance we take toward ourselves and the world.

Learning how to observe the mechanism involved in breathing, as well as the various physical, emotional and mental forces acting on them, depends in large part on learning how to sense ourselves, to listen to ourselves, to expand our attention to include the sensory impressions constantly arising in our organism. We have to learn to listen to our body.

You Can if You Think You Can

IF YOU HAVE A WELLNESS problem, now or in the future, you come to the realization something needs to be done. Maybe it's obesity, vascular disease with strokes and heart attacks, or type 2 diabetes. Don't feel hopeless or give up, do something about it. Anything is possible. Even if it's advanced cancer, positive thinking and mind-body techniques can double your lifespan and increase spontaneous cure rate—based to my own experience and what I read in the literature. Cancer specialists as a group are just too pessimistic. There are so many books on the subject. They fill my library, books on hope and what to do.

When you have a problem, one that is especially difficult and baffling, perhaps unendurable and discouraging, there is one basic principle—never quit. To do so is to admit defeat and your defeatist attitude will come true. Giving up shows a defective personality. It tends to develop a defeatist psychology.

Come at the problem in a different way if the methodology you're using is not working. And if the new approach is not working, come at it another way until you find the key. The computer button that turns on the human brain, your mind, remembers what it is like to be well. Be persistent, it's always too soon to quit.

How do you develop this undefeatable attitude? You need to develop a program of hope. Throw hopelessness out the window. Don't talk yourself into defeat. It is dangerous to use negative words. No, denotes that you shut the door. It means defeat it delays improvement. Turn things around, and now you have more. Meet the problem. Change your thinking; meet the problem in a positive, constant optimistic way. Make a plan; write it down. It's motivating.

The refusal to quit is called the persistence principle. Perseverance will win the day—don't be quitters. Send out your positive vision, you cannot create success anywhere in this life without this application of the persistence principle.

Keep thinking positively. Much rain wears down marble. I saw that myself at St. Peter's Cathedral in Rome. If you don't first succeed, then try again. The Perception of all of yourself is critical and is applied by the perseverance principle.

Many times we are our own worst enemy. People can have goals and objectives and work hard and still fail. Perhaps you need to look at yourself and something is amiss in yourself. Sharing what you think may be your personality defects with another person, almost any person, can be of great value. Especially if you bring spirituality into it. Remember attending church is the path to spirituality, no matter what religion.

The hardest person to know is yourself. We have a built-in self-protecting mechanism that always tries to do what we want. It seeks to make the irrational appear rational. Many people will talk about other people and their problems, but they hide from themselves and their own problems.

People who failed usually do that, not because they unable to handle another situation—this is just in conflict with what they've been doing. Remember, if you're doing the same thing again and again, don't expect a different outcome.

You must see yourself as you really are and deal with yourself on that honest basis. That is the perception concept. And it is based on self-examination, a realistic look at yourself because you're nearing the end of the road, or just traveling on the road of poor health and lack of wellness. Stand in front of a mirror and say to yourself, "Now I want the truth about you."

The normal person will realize that self-knowledge is always a beginning of self-development. The process is motivated by perception and releases new powers. It is the road that leads to successful achievement. Plugging away will win the day. Problems are a sign of life. Success weakens you; problem solving strengthens you.

How do you solve a problem, and get motivated to solve the problem? If you acknowledge of the problem, and apply thought and belief, then you have taken a long step down the road to handling it successfully.

Study your health problem; read about it; attend my free lectures; become knowledgeable; then find the weak spot. Break the problem apart, and the rest will be easy. We need the body to carry the brain around. The mind is you. The tendency is to react emotionally rather than to think. The human mind will not think properly when it is hot. Cool it when problems start. Make use of your spiritual power. You can if you think you can, because all the ideas you need to handle every problem are all about you. Cool reactions will open up the lines of communication by which ideas flow to you. The chief duty of a human being is to master life.

To be healthy, vital, and alive, it is very important how you think. To a degree you can think yourself sick, or you could think yourself well. The soul becomes dyed with the color of its thoughts. If you think unhealthy, you will become unhealthy. Think defeat and you will tend to create the circumstances that lead to defeat. You can if you think you can. In the matter of well being, positive results come from visualizing yourself as whole, and you will act on it and get it done.

Love is the Answer

WHEN YOU'RE TALKING ABOUT HEALTH, love has a lot to do with it. Let's face it, if you're trying to attract or get the attention of another person, getting in shape and looking good works a lot of the time. If you don't take care of yourself, you certainly are less likely to be found attractive by another individual. Are you overweight? Do you smell like cigarettes? Don't discount the power of love. If you're harboring feelings of anger, anxiety or lack self-esteem, this negative way of thinking could be eating away at your immune system and your health. Your immune system feels what you feel. If your body feels love, it is much more likely to heal. Love of another person, a family, or group can lead to healing. I personally have seen it many times in my 41 years of practicing medicine. Love is a vast and open-ended sensation, the most written about, talked about, and worried about emotion in the history of humankind and can be expressed in countless ways.

Love can be love of nature. It can mean you feel oneness with the universe. It gives us a warm, fuzzy emotion you have been doing something as simple as appreciating a cozy fireplace or watching a movie with your loved one, or the warm sensation when you hug someone. Love is the sense of appreciation, understanding, sympathy, and empathy. It expresses connection, whether it is to a family member or just a friend, or even a perfect stranger.

Love is the antidote to hate, anger, fear and sadness. Your 70 trillion cells feel good when you feel love. Your 70 trillion body cells feel pain when you lead a life without love. Our immune system is very attuned to our feelings.

It has been proved scientifically that negative thinking and emotions accelerate aging and cause heart disease, cancer and inflammatory diseases. The studies were published in the American Medical Association Journal. It is well known that happy people are healthier. Happy people live longer with cancer, and the spontaneous cure rate goes up. That is well publicized in medical literature. If we experienced love of life, the longer we will live and be more protected against a lot of diseases of aging.

Love can be defined as an inner peace, an attitude that can arise from faith, from a spiritual belief system, and the rewards are plentiful. Married people live longer; a person living in isolation has a lot more illness and dies a lot sooner. We all know that, many times after the death of a spouse, the survivor may die within a year or 2.

The love of nature has a lot of healing properties. Look what a walk in the park or woods can do for you. It's rejuvenating. I speak to the animals and flowers and find it exhilarating. A walk down a city street will also do that for you. One of the most extraordinary kinds of love is an appreciation for the wonder of nature and for the awesome interconnections between all the facets of the world. Just walking in a quiet rain or early snow can be very rejuvenating. Once when sitting in a tree, observing nature and watching the day go by—I don't hunt—the dew started falling from the leaves, the sun started rising, it was heavenly. Little droplets of water, falling out of the sky, bringing dew on all the grass, plants and trees can get you to fall in love with nature and has many healing properties. How can you not feel love for nature? It can be very motivating to wellness.

There are countless ways to feel love. When you're with someone, it can be a hug, a touch, or look. Just to say "I love you" can be very healing and motivate you to wellness. Interpersonal love heals. Lovers live longer; that has been scientifically proven. People who are in painful relationships have more illnesses and die sooner and develop bad health habits because of the stress. We all have heard of the broken-heart syndrome "stress cardio-myopathy". Sudden emotional stress can put you in the intensive care unit, be life-threatening, and can cause changes in your EKG, shortness of breath, and even heart failure. Yet, no changes are found on the angiogram. Most of these people do recover. Being in a high-quality relationship has been found to be protective for the heart.

Don't forget to love yourself, which can be most difficult if what you are doing is not consistent with the image of yourself. That's the biggest cause of stress. The inability to cope with threats, real or imaginary, to our emotional, physical, and spiritual being, is the best definition of stress. We all want to be happy, we want to be loved, and we want to love others. That is motivational and healing. Social connectedness improves health and longevity, and social isolation increases mortality. Love is motivating, hate and anger, demotivating. I can clearly tell when treating my patients, by checking the social history—the amount of family love they are exposed to—what the odds of that person healing themselves are. Isolated people don't do well. Let your currency be love and happiness. Be a happy person and say loving things to other people. Leave notes of love around the house, the community around you will send you love in return. That's healing.

Dr. Mark Liponis, the medical director of the Canyon Ranch in Arizona and Massachusetts, calls love vitamin L. He states, often his patients have so much money, freedom, good jobs, fancy homes, but they lack the most important asset—love. I found that recently in a neighbor of mine in Naples Florida. He lives in the fanciest place I ever did see, but I felt sorry for him. He lived there by himself for months at a time, while his wife was back home in Chicago. She went around the world last year by herself on a 747 Jet. How sad, he did not have good health and complained of being lonely. Well, I now have a new friend, who I will be inviting to go to dinner with my wife and me when I get back to Florida next week. With little love in your life, the need for food can be de-motivating and not healthy for you. It takes a lifetime of work to be loving, but we can always get better. Even if love is atrophied, it can be revived and renewed, as long as you want to restore it.

Dr. Mark Liponis has a number of recommendations. Tell someone you love him or her, get a pet, keep a love journal, read some books. On page 173 of his book, *Ultra Longevity*, he lists a number of books, you can read. One that he recommends is *The Art of happiness: a Handbook for Living* by the Dalai Lama. He also recommends watching some loving and funny movies, using a love mantra like the one I plan to use, and he recommends "All You Need Is Love" by the Beatles.

Lennon/McCartney

Love, love, love, love, love, love, love, love, love.
There's nothing you can do that can't be done.
Nothing you can sing that can't be sung.
Nothing you can say but you can learn how to play the game
It's easy.

There's nothing you can make that can't be made.
No one you can save that can't be saved.
Nothing you can do but you can learn how to be you
In time - It's easy.
All you need is love, all you need is love,
All you need is love, love, love is all you need.
Love, love, love, love, love, love, love, love, love.
All you need is love, all you need is love,
All you need is love, love, love is all you need.
There's nothing you can know that isn't known.
Nothing you can see that isn't shown.
Nowhere you can be that isn't where you're meant to be.
It's easy.
All you need is love, all you need is love,
All you need is love, love, love is all you need.
All you need is love (all together now)
All you need is love (everybody)
All you need is love, love, love is all you need.

Let's get to work. There can be great benefits and bring love into your life. It will motivate you to happiness, a long life, a lot of energy, and very little sickness.

Keep It Simple

THE FOLLOWING TIPS WILL MAKE it simple for you to eat and live well:

1) Make a commitment.
2) Use a mantra — empowering words that inspire you such as -"I want to live to be hundred without disease, look good, honor my god or spirit."
3) Visualize the result daily: Make a mental picture of how you want to look and feel.
4) Educate yourself and participate in your healthcare.
5) Motivate yourself with a friend or a small group of friends who are also committed to a healthy lifestyle.
6) Keep a food journal for at least 3 to 6 months, until your new healthy ways are a habit.
7) Think about what you are about to eat 5 minutes before your meal so you make more conscious choices.
8) Place a sign on your refrigerator, which says, "If I'm not hungry, I don't eat."
9) Avoid eating after 7 p.m.
10) Clean all of the sugary products out of your kitchen.
11) Have at least 5 sugarless snacks available for travel, work and home.
12) Learn to cook and teach your kids how to cook.

General Plan
1) No sugary drinks, no diet drinks
2) 6 to 8 glasses of water daily
3) 30-50% less fructose
4) No more than 2-3 pieces of fruit daily
5) 50%vegetables, 25% of 100% complex carbs, 25% lean organic meat, nuts and seeds
6) Detox for 2 weeks
7) Exercise for 30 minutes 5 days a week, lift weights 3 days a week
8) Avoid dairy products
9) Avoid wheat if gluten sensitive

Rules
1) If it has a label, don't eat it (or at least learn to read the label).
2) Avoid food in a box or package
3) Don't add salt
4) Stay away from deadly white flour and sugar products
5) Know the fructose content of your food-see table back of the book
6) Avoid any food that has high fructose corn syrup in it
7) Avoid all sweeteners
8) No diet drinks
9) Throw out any food with preservatives, additives, coloring or dies or natural flavors like MSG.
10) Eat organic foods without hormones, pesticides and other chemicals.
11) Lean meat or fish should be organic-not from a pond or from concentrated animal feeding organizations.
12) Use only plant oils sparingly olive or coconut oil.

13) Increase intake of dark, green, leafy vegetables, including spinach, collard greens, turnip greens, mustard greens, vegetables that grow in the ground, cabbage, green beans, squash, cauliflower, onions, mushrooms.

14) Limited intake of saturated fat and primarily use mono saturated fats, olives, avocados, nuts and seeds. Eliminate animal products (meat and dairy).

15) Eat fruit low on the glycemic index, 2 to 3 pieces daily at most.

16) Limit fructose intake to around 35 grams daily.

Enjoy the following foods:
non-starchy veggies-low glycemic index foods
asparagus
bell peppers
broccoli
cauliflower
collard greens
cucumbers
green beans
kale
spinach
zucchini
Proteins:
beans
chicken
eggs
fish
lentils
nuts
seeds

turkey
Starchy foods:
Beets
brown or black rice
carrots
buckwheat
corn
quinoa
sweet potatoes
turnips
winter squash
Low glycemic fruit:
apples
blackberries
blueberries
gogi berries
plums
kiwi
nectarines
peaches
raspberries
fruits with stones (seeds)

The Secrets

FOLLOWING ARE SEVERAL SECRETS TO a healthy diet and lifestyle that will help you along the way:

1) All carbohydrates are not alike. Starchy, complex carbohydrates quell hunger and turn up our internal furnace, burning calories as heat and energy. High sugar, high fat, simple carbohydrates increase hunger, food addictions and cravings.

2) The same starchy carbohydrates that prevent disease and premature death stop and even reverse disease.

3) The resistant starch in complex carbohydrates absorbs fat and cholesterol, while providing few calories and the feeling of fullness.

4) Refined carbohydrates reduce the "good" HDL cholesterol and increase insulin levels, triglycerides, blood pressure and fat stores-proven culprits in the development of inflammation, obesity, and diabetes and vascular disease.

5) Foods that promote weight loss are high in complex carbohydrates, which take more energy, calories, to break down. A faster metabolism and burn excess body fat.

6) Consumption of complex carbohydrates helps the brain produce higher levels of serotonin, which reduces your appetite and increases your feelings of well-being.

7) Reducing saturated fat without reducing refined carbo-hydrates works against the goal to lose weight and pre-vent or reverse chronic disease.

8) Saturated fats increase water clogging LDL cholesterol. The unsaturated fats and fish, flax seeds and plant-based oils reduce LDL cholesterol, inflammation and plaque within blood vessels.

9) Trans fat offer what the Mayo Clinic calls "a cholesterol double whammy" by raising "bad" LDL-cholesterol and lowering "good" HDL-cholesterol. The greater the per-centage of trans fat in a food product, the higher risk for heart attacks and strokes.

10) Try to limit olive and other cooking oils while trying to lose weight, and then use them sparingly. Fish, ground flax seeds and walnuts offer the benefits of omega-3 fatty acids without all the fat of oil.

11) Animal protein raises cholesterol while plant protein low-ers it. Meat also raises it.

12) To get the mental amount of protein you need each day, balance your vegetables with legumes and some nuts.

13) To lose weight faster, choose raw foods such as apples, carrots, bell peppers and other whole foods and vegeta-bles eaten raw. Snacking on crunchy foods slows the rate of digestion and provides thousands of disease-fighting nutrients.

14) It takes 30 to 40 calories a day to maintain one pound of muscle. The more lean body mass you have, the faster your metabolism will be, and the greater number of cal-ories you burn at rest. Do some weight training every week.

15) The same starchy carbohydrates that promote weight loss can prevent, stop and even reverse disease.
16) Eat a diet of foods containing vitamins, minerals and phytochemicals; it is the rainbow, symphony and mosaic of these that leads to good health.

MORE RESOURCES FROM RUDY KACHMANN M.D.

Also visit Dr. Kachmann's YouTube channel www.youtube.com/drrudykachmann

Books:
Our Body On Fire
Fructose – The Evil Twin
The Golden Opportunity
Narcotics: The Highway To Hell
Pain: We Need a New Definition
The Fraud of Chronic Pain
Healing Cancer with The Power Of Your Mind
Live to Be 100 with a Sound Mind and Body
The Call of Life
The Fraud of Alzheimer's Disease
Nocebo: Placebo's Evil Twin
The Secret of the Non Diet for Adults
The Secret of the Non Diet for Children
Kid Scripts: Just What the Doctor Ordered
The Psychology of Eating
Reversing Type 2
Welcome to Your Mind Body
Secrets of Motivating Yourself to Wellness

Available at: www.amazon.com and other retailers
www.youtube.com/drrudykachmann

www.ingramcontent.com/pod-product-compliance
Lightning Source LLC
Chambersburg PA
CBHW060249290526
45789CB00001B/258